No-Drama Appro
[3 in 1]

How to Make the Potty Experience Fun and Easy for Your Child

By

MISSY RHYMES

Table of Contents

Potty Training in A Weekend

Potty Training for Newborn Superheroes

Time-Saving Potty Training

Potty Training in A Weekend

The Step-By-Step Guide to Potty Train Your Little Toddler in Less Than 3 Days. Perfect for Little Boys and Girls. Bonus Chapter with Tips for Careless Dads Included

MISSY RHYMES

Table of Contents

Introduction

Congratulations on purchasing <u>Potty Training in A Weekend</u>: The Step-By-Step Guide to Potty Train Your Little Toddler in Less Than 3 Days. Perfect for Little Boys and Girls. Bonus Chapter with Tips for Careless Dads Included and thank you for doing so.

The following chapters will discuss the step-by-step instructions to potty train your child in just three days. Going beyond the bare minimum, this book covers not only just the physical steps that will need to be taken but also the mental preparation that will ensure that both you and your child are set up for success! This book will dispel the myths and misconceptions surrounding the potty training process and will outline how parents and caregivers can use psychology to make the potty training process more teamwork and less brute force. By following the system outlined here, potty training will be a shared goal that both parents and/or caregivers and their children will want to achieve together!

Not only will parents and caregivers benefit from learning how to create a spirit of teamwork during the process, but parents and caregivers will also learn how

to handle the potty training outliers when potty training is not going as it should. Learning how to best support children in a variety of scenarios is an important part of potty training successfully and in a healthy manner.

To set the reader of this book up for success, it is important to begin with a strong knowledge base of the physiological and psychological processes behind potty training, or potty learning from the child's perspective. In other words, parents and caregivers need to know the physical and emotional processes at work during this period of time in order to best support their children through it. A brief note to the reader: Be prepared to hear some "potty talk" in this book! It is both necessary and healthy to be able to use accurate bathroom-related terminology during this process. Ultimately you will choose what terminology you use with your child, but for the purposes of this book it will be important to use bathroom-related language, so be prepared.

In addition to the real-life advice found throughout this book, there is also a bonus chapter that includes potty training tips and tricks from real-life dads fordads still in the trenches! All too often, books aimed at parents and caregivers forget that fathers are an Important

part of this team, and the unique relationship they have with their children can be utilized in specific endeavors like this for ultimate success for everyone.

There are plenty of books on this subject on the market, thanks again for choosing this one! Every effort was made to ensure it is full of as much useful information as possible, please enjoy it!

Chapter 1: In the Beginning

As you prepare yourself to begin the process of potty training with your child, there are techniques that you can use to prepare both yourself and your child to set yourselves up for ultimate success during this process! A significant part of this preparation will be the mental preparation because the mindset that both you and your child enter into this endeavor with will largely determine how quickly you are successful. The process of preparing yourself and your child mentally for the new journey you are undertaking is called priming, and it is going to play a huge part in helping your potty training process run smoothly.

To begin, you must prime yourself to approach potty training in a healthy and practical manner. Sadly, according to the American Academy of Pediatrics, the premier children's health governing body in the United States of America, the developmental experience that has the most potential for abuse of children is potty training and it is easy to imagine why. Frustrations are understandable during potty training as pressure is high for everyone: parents, caregivers, and trainees! It will be important that parents and caregivers

understand how to best manage their expectations and any frustrations that may come up during the process.

Parents and caregivers are understandably anxious during the potty training process as there is truly only so much that a parent or caregiver can do. It is always ultimately up to the child if they are ready to ditch their diapers or not, and this is not likely an intentional choice on the part of the child as much as it is just the result of their developmental reality at that moment.

In addition to this, parents and caregivers are also under the additional burden of the actual work involved in potty training. While most parents and caregivers are more than ready to shuck the diapers to the curb for the additional ease and freedom of having a toilet-trained child, the reality is that there will be much more work coming down the pike before the child is fully potty trained. Before the child is fully potty trained, there will be plenty of accidents and additional laundry, as well as the extra mental and physical work of setting timers and organizing and developing a game plan that involves potty schedules and schematics for rewards and reinforcement!

Children feed off of this anxiety and pressure as they

often recognize the importance of this monumental task being placed in front of them. This has the potential to create power struggles around toilet use, and nobody wants that! It is understandable that children will act out and push back against this pressure and anxiety, and this is what can lead to unacceptable and even dangerous uses of force from parents and caregivers as unnecessary and unproductive punishments intended to manipulate their children's behavior.

Careful examination of the expectations that parents and caregivers hold over their children's capabilities as well as a solid game plan to complete the potty training process will help to set the parent and/or caregiver up for success with their children.

Some of the expectations that parents and caregivers hold around the potty training process are a result of myths and misconceptions around the practice that have been around for many, many years that we will cover now.

Myth #1

There is a magic potty training age that if a parent and/or caregiver begins, the child will be more successful in the potty training process.

Fact

Every child develops according to their own schedule! Potty training is not an exact science because every child will have their own distinctly unique timetable as to when their mind and body is ready will be ready to begin the process. There is no need to put extra pressure on the process by ignoring the signs and signals your child is showing you as to whether or not they are ready to begin potty training just because the calendar says so!

Most children potty train sometime between the ages of two and four, with outliers that begin younger than two and those that are still training beyond the age of four.

Myth #2

Potty training is something parents do to and for their children, not with their children.

Fact

This is as wrong as wrong can be! Potty training is not something that a parent and/or caregiver can do for their child, it is an interactive process that requires cooperation and teamwork from both parent and/or caregiver and child. You want your child to be your

partner in this venture!

Myth #3

Your child is being willfully disobedient if they won't potty train according to your schedule and expectations.

Fact

While it could be true that your child is willfully pushing potty training away, this does not necessarily mean that your child is being disobedient. As was discussed in the introduction, there are many reasons why you cannot force a child to potty train before they are ready. There are physical and mental processes that must be developed before a child can fully learn the skill of proper toilet use.

Myth #4

If you've already potty trained an older sibling using a specific method, then the younger siblings should also be able to train using that method.

Fact

Each child is their own unique and individualistic person with their own personal needs and capabilities. Each child develops in their own time and what may have worked for their older sibling (or their cousin, or neighbor, or playmate) may not necessarily work for them.

Myth #5

Once my child potty trains, there is no looking back!

Fact

This is a very common myth. It is not accurate, however. Most children do go on to have accidents for some time after potty training. The window for becoming a potty pro is quite wide for small children, with some children having accidents up to a few years after they officially "potty train" and ditch their diapers. This is very normal. There is much to distract small children and it can be very easy to forget all about their bodily functions when they are learning so much every day about this dazzling new world all around them!

Myth #6

If we potty train our child to use the toilet during the day, we should potty train our child to stay dry throughout the night, too.

Fact

There are schools of thought regarding potty training that believe that potty training should be an "all or nothing" sort of experience, and this includes getting rid of any sort of diaper or pull-up type of training pants at nighttime. However, potty training at night is actually a completely different process than the process for potty training during the day because a child's ability to stay dry throughout the night has less to do with learning proper toileting habits and bodily signals and more to do with night time hormones related to urine production and the degree to how heavily your child sleeps. Most doctors and urologists agree that nighttime bladder control is not an issue until the child is around seven years old.

As you can see, there are many myths and misconceptions surrounding the potty training experience that can set a parent and/or caregiver up for expectations that can't be met. Sometimes this is a result of failing to recognize what potty learning truly is for the child.

For a child that has been diapered since birth, learning how to ditch their diapers requires a whole world of

complexity that parents and caregivers often do not take the time to consider. For their tiny little bodies and minds, they have never had to pay much attention to their elimination habits. They've always just had their waste products exit their bodies when it needed to, without any real consideration or effort on their parts. To begin the potty training process, parents and caregivers must realize that they are essentially starting from scratch!

The child must first learn to be aware of her body and its functions. This requires an awareness that what is consumed will need to then exit the body as a waste product eventually. For some children, this is a surprise! Taking the time to help teach them this connection is an important building block in the potty training process. They need to understand that the juice box they just drank will be ready to come out within the next hour or so, and this will be an important part of the methodology in Chapter 2 when you are introduced to the steps of the three-day potty training method.

In addition to being aware that what comes in must go out, children must then learn to be aware of what it

feels like *before* they need the toilet. Again, they have never needed to be aware of the sensation of a full bladder in need of emptying in their life, their bodies have just released whenever they needed to without any help or awareness on the part of the child. This process of paying attention to the body and learning to associate the sensations of their body with the need to sit on the potty chair is often one of the most aggravating aspects of potty training for both the child and their parents and/or caregivers.

One way to facilitate your child's learning about their bodily functions and the awareness of when they need to visit the restroom is to model this for them with your actions. This would include announcing to your child when you need to use the restroom and using descriptive language that they will understand. You will know your child best, but this could sound something like, "Oh, I think that glass of water I just drank is ready to come out! My bladder feels full, I need to pee/urinate/whatever terminology you choose," and you would say this while perhaps poking one finger into your lower abdomen over your bladder. Or perhaps you might say, "Oh, my stomach hurts a little bit down here,

I need to poop/defecate/whatever terminology you choose," and you would also say this while motioning to your lower abdomen. The point here is to help your child learn where these parts of their body are so they can begin to associate these areas with making a trip to the potty. You are also teaching them the language they will need during their potty training experience.

The other crucial element here is in modeling the actual process for our children. Children are visual creatures, and they love to do what they see others doing! For most children, their primary caregivers and/or parents are their primary models of behavior and being allowed to see a parent and/or caregiver sit on the toilet and go through the process themselves can give them a clear example of how they're supposed to do it. It is also important here to narrate the process for your little one, like this: "Okay, I have to pee now so I'm going to the potty. I'm going to pull my shorts down and sit here on the potty. Okay…. Now I just need to let my pee out! There it is, can you hear it? That's my pee going into the toilet! Alright, now I can grab a little bit of toilet paper, just like this, and wipe myself clean. Now I just need to toss it in the potty, pull my shorts back up, and

flush! Ready to hear the toilet flush? Here it goes and WOO! Alright, now I get to wash my hands! I like this soap, it's blue. Pretty cool, right?"

Notice in the narrative above that the parent and/or caregiver is not only narrating each part of the experience, but they are also making the entire experience sound like fun! Children will want to also be able to mimic this experience, especially aspects like flushing the toilet. The entire experience needs to be described like it is something that is a great part of growing up. This is a part of priming the experience for your child. If the experience is primed as something fun and attractive, your child will join you in this quest rather than resist you.

In addition to this physical learning about the parts of your child's body and their awareness of them and what they do, there is a cognitive aspect that is required in potty training. Children must be able to not only feel the sensation of a full bladder or a bowel movement, but they must also be able to reason and rationalize with themselves to a certain extent. Young children often struggle with this part of the potty training process because it can be difficult for them to

understand and engage in delayed gratification or time awareness. If a child is playing with their favorite toy in the living room, it won't matter too much if they feel the pressure of a full bladder and understand what that means if they don't have the cognitive skills yet to understand that they can set the toy down to go to the restroom and then come back for the toy again. For young children, they live in the moment, every moment. This cognitive awareness is one of the most crucial aspects of potty training and one of the reasons why so many of the "potty training tips and tricks" geared towards young toddlers do not work. A very young toddler simply will not have this cognitive awareness down enough to be able to make this choice, and this can lead to serious bladder and bodily issues when they are trained to hold their waste anyway.

This is why pediatrician and urologist groups caution against enforcing any potty training protocol before a child is displaying at least the following signs of readiness: able to communicate their need to use the toilet either verbally or nonverbally, can physically get themselves to the restroom safely and efficiently by either walking or crawling, can dress and undress themselves to use the toilet, and can sit safely on a

toilet seat unassisted. Enforcing a potty training program before a child is ready can result in urinary tract infections, kidney damage, constipation, and a lifetime of poor toileting habits.

Parents and caregivers can assess if their child is cognitively prepared to begin the potty training process by gauging how much interest and self-awareness the child has around all things potty related. Ask yourself the following questions to see if your little one is cognitively prepared for potty training!

- Does your child express interest in the toilet by following family members into the restroom or commenting on "going potty" when it is mentioned?

- Does your child express interest in "being a big kid" and want to do what older siblings and older children do?

- Does your child express when their diaper is soiled by pulling on the wet/dirty diaper, trying to remove it or even removing it themselves, and/or announcing that they need a diaper change?

If you answered yes to all three of these questions, then

it is very likely that your child is cognitively prepared to begin the potty training process! Ask yourself the following questions to see if your little one is physically prepared for potty training!

- Is your child able to verbally and nonverbally express their physical needs, such as by asking for something to drink when thirsty or by stating they are cold and need a sweater?

- Is your child able to physically get themselves, without assistance, to the toilet and back by crawling or walking?

- Is your child able to dress and undress themselves efficiently enough to do so in the restroom largely unassisted?

- Is your child able to safely sit unassisted on a toilet or potty chair?

If you answered yes to all of these questions, then it is very likely that your child is physically prepared to begin the potty training process!

Once your child is demonstrating the cognitive and physical signs of readiness for potty training, then you can safely move on to the three-day potty training

system! But first, a few words on the mental preparation moving forward.

You and your child will need to be a team in this endeavor. Not only is this necessary because one person cannot force another person to use a toilet (not safely and respectfully, anyway!) but it is also a matter of simple psychology.

Toddlers want to please their parents and caregivers- although it may not always seem like it! This perception happens because, for so much of those early childhood years, children have little to no bodily autonomy or control over where they go or what they do. This leaves them very few opportunities to assert their independence and capabilities in a healthy and constructive manner. This often translates then to what adults often view as being "petty" demands and tantrums, such as may occur over what color cup the child wants to drink out of or whether the child wants to put on their shoes or not.

Step back a moment and try to look at it from this tiny person's perspective for a moment: If you had no control over what time you woke up in the morning, what you had available to eat, no capabilities to perform

the majority of the tasks being performed around you (cooking, driving, talking on the phone, etc) and little to no choice over how you spend your days, wouldn't you also on occasion feel the need to make a choice of your own, on your own terms, no matter how trivial it may seem to others? This is the perspective of the small child, and the more that parents and caregivers can explore and understand this, the better they will be able to work with their child's psychology so that everyone can experience a win.

This is where the psychology behind team building comes in. Parents and caregivers don't need the potty training process to be any more difficult than what it already will be and should take all the help they can get! This includes the help of their small child, and it begins with how the child is approached with the process of potty training.

The child should never be made to feel as if potty training is an event that is coming up that they will be forced to be a part of, but rather should feel as if they are making the decision to begin potty training. This is easy enough to do for most children between the ages of two and four because this age range is typically in

the "I want to do it all by myself" mentality as they are looking to develop more of the autonomy and independence, they see being exercised by older people around them.

A note to parents and caregivers on how they speak to one another about the potty training process: Watch how you are wording your conversations within earshot of your small child. Keep in mind that children are almost always listening, even when they appear busy at play.

Comments that may not seem like much of a big deal can play into negative perspectives about the potty training process when heard by young ears that don't entirely understand what it all means. An example of this might sound something like, "We plan on <voice dropping conspiratorially> *potty training* this weekend," or "I just hope it's nothing like <insert name of child's playmate here> because their mom told me it was absolutely miserable! They spent months fighting it." This is even more of an issue for those comments that are made between parents and caregivers where there is visible negative body language such as head shaking, eye-rolling, or whispering behind hands.

Children are more aware of these social cues than parents and caregivers often assume, and this is not a good way to prime the potty training experience for your child!

In the interest of setting up the experience of potty training as a shared goal and shared effort, look around for examples of meaningful models that your child may use for potty training. Is there an older sibling that they look up to? Is there maybe an older neighbor that is close to the family? Or perhaps a favorite cartoon character?

Remember, you want your child to *want* to potty train, otherwise, it will be you trying to *force* your child to complete this developmental process, and this rarely works. Think about other developmental leaps that children take such as crawling, walking, and even talking. Has any parent and/or caregiver ever succeeded in forcing a baby to crawl? Is there any physical way to force a baby to walk when they simply don't have the leg and core strength and coordination between their body parts? How about forcing a baby to walk that simply doesn't have any interest in it yet because they still prefer to crawl? No, of course not.

Just as we encourage our children to learn to talk by modeling it for them and engaging with them verbally in a fun way, we can do the same with the developmental process of potty training.

Keeping this in mind, enlist the help of the meaningful models that you know your child will look up to and want to emulate. If it is an older sibling, ask the older sibling to join in on the modeling of bathroom behavior by both physically modeling the process and narrating in a fun and upbeat way. The older sibling can even say things like, "someday you will be able to do the potty just like me! Isn't that cool?"

If your child's meaningful model is a neighbor, you can ask the neighbor to announce before they have to run to the restroom, saying in an excited voice, "I have to go to the potty now, I'll be right back to keep playing with you in just a moment!" This would model both the process of making the decision to go to the toilet and also the idea that you can take a quick break from playing to go to the restroom and come right back to it.

If your child's meaningful model is a beloved cartoon character, then use that! There are a variety of ways that you can make this happen. There are many cartoon

character toys that demonstrate the potty process and even sing cute little songs about going to the restroom, and they are available from major retailers; a quick google search will reveal what is available in that department.

There are also several cartoon episodes dedicated to teaching children how to go to the potty, and these are available in many different streaming services such as Netflix, Hulu, Amazon Prime, and PBS Kids, to name a few. They are also largely available via a quick google search, so do take advantage of that!

One children's show that is renowned for its successful induction of children into the potty training experience is PBS Kids' Daniel Tiger's Neighborhood and their episode, "Daniel Goes to the Potty." This episode features the beloved main character, Daniel Tiger, learning to go sit on the potty. The song that Daniel sings every time he feels the urge to go to the potty is incredibly catchy and memorable and has been used successfully by many a parent and caregiver to remind a child that they need to go sit on the potty!

If you are a screen-free family and have no interest in using media to help during the potty training process,

then feel free to be creative and make up your own potty training song for your little one to sing! The catchier, the better. Make it something fun and upbeat that your child and you enjoy singing every time they need to go sit on the potty. This is a part of keeping the experience fun and upbeat. It's amazing what our children will do in pursuit of light-hearted fun with their parents and caregivers!

To further prime the potty training experience for your child, you can determine how to best set up your restroom for your child. Many parents and caregivers choose to use an independent potty chair, which is the small, child-size potty that can be purchased at any major retailer/big box store or online. An advantage of this is the safety feature of it being their perfect size and situated firmly on the ground. There is also a feeling of pride in ownership that many children feel when they have their very own little potty, just for them to use. Some parents even take their children with them to the store to pick out their very own potty chair or give them stickers to decorate the potty chair and make it their own.

Another option is to purchase one of the seat modifiers

that are also available through any major retailer and big box store or online that either attaches to the regular toilet seat or can be easily placed on top that makes the toilet seat a more child-friendly size. There are a few advantages to this, such as if bathroom space is limited and there is simply no room for another potty chair in the same room. Some children even prefer this option over the standalone child-size potty chair because they feel like more of a "big kid" with this option, and this seems to be the case more often when there is an older sibling as the child's meaningful model.

Another option that is similar to the seat modifier is to simply add a safety stool for the child so they can more easily get up on the regular toilet themselves. Often times this option can even be found with a hand-rail so they have something to keep their balance while climbing on and off. An advantage of this particular option is that it fulfills the same desire of the child to feel like a "big kid" in using the regular potty, and it also teaches them the necessary skills to navigate the regular-sized toilets they will find outside of the home. This can be very helpful for some children that may be uneasy about moving from the child-size options at

home to the regular size toilets that they will find while using the restroom outside of the home.

Whatever potty option you choose, be sure to tailor it to your child and their needs. If you know that doing it "just like the big kids do" is going to be a big motivator, then perhaps it might be best to go with the options that modify the standard size toilet. If you know that your child doesn't like sitting on full-size chairs as well as smaller child-size chairs, then perhaps the child-size potty chair is best. If you know your child is always excited to sit in regular-sized chairs to be "like a big kid" then using the regular toilet with a safety addition might be the right incentive for them.

Your shopping trip also needs to include some favorite beverage options for your child. This is important because you will need to have your child drinking plenty of fluids during the three-day potty training weekend. This is to ensure that your child is experiencing a full bladder and the sensations that come along with it as you teach your child to associate that sensation with the need to go sit on the toilet. Parents often opt for both regular favorites and "special" beverages that the child rarely gets so there will be no question as to if the child will be interested in drinking them. You know your child best, but fruit juices, lemonades, or any sort of sweet beverage is usually always a hit with any small child!

The next thing to gather in preparation for your three-day potty training process is the underwear that your child will be replacing their diapers with! Many children really get a kick out of picking out their "big kid" underwear, so take them shopping with you. This also plays into the pride of ownership psychology, in which you want your child to feel like they have some control here, too. Really have fun with this, talk it up at the store and make it exciting and fun to get to pick out underwear with their favorite characters, colors, and patterns on them. Remember, this is all a part of priming the experience for your child!

Pro tip from a parent that has been there, done that: However, many pairs you think you need to start off with, double it. At the very least, double it! It is very likely that you will need them- and then some- during your potty training weekend extravaganza, so prep yourself well here!

Another important shopping trip that must take place

before the three-day potty training process is the trip in which you procure the treats and rewards that you will use to keep your child associating potty use with celebration and reward. Parents and caregivers will know their children best, but whatever you do, diversify your treat and reward supplies!

Some common ideas for treats and rewards that are often used during the potty training process are small candies such as skittles, smarties, or M&Ms that allow for sweet, exciting treats to be doled out just a couple at a time. Stickers with favorite cartoon and storybook characters on them and little puzzle and workbook-style books that your child can interact with are always a big hit! Some parents and caregivers like to create a treasure box of sorts for the potty training experience that the child gets to pick out after they've had a successful trip to the potty, and this is often filled with a variety of sweet treats and small prize style toys. Dollar stores often provide a great value for this avenue, as you can buy many little exciting "treasures" for the child that won't break the bank! Anything that is new and different is typically enough to incentivize a child to want to participate in the potty training process so they can earn their rewards!

Some parents and caregivers choose to share the treasure box with the child the day before the potty training process kicks off by letting the child take a peek and know that tomorrow, they will get a chance to check it out and pick items out for themselves when they use the big-kid potty. This gives them an element of excitement to associate with the big day!

Before the child heads off to bed the night before the potty training weekend, you can let them know that tomorrow you will be throwing away the diaper they are wearing and they will get to wear their big kid underwear and try the big kid potty! Let them know they will get to pick prizes out of the treasure box every time they pee or poop on their potty and that you will be right there with them to celebrate with them. Make sure they hear that you are excited for the next day and you are confident that you guys will have a great day. Let your child drift off to sleep imagining the exciting things awaiting them the next day!

In order to successfully utilize the Potty Training in A Weekend methodology, it is important to have a three-day long weekend devoted exclusively to the potty training process. This means that there need to be

three days dedicated to the potty training process. No trips to the park, no running to the grocery store, no guests in the house to distract the parent and/or caregiver, and if you can swing it, siblings either 100% on board with helping be a part of this process or spending the long weekend out at a friend's house. The only thing you and your child should be doing over the course of this three-day weekend will be sharing this potty training experience!

Parents and caregivers that have been there and done that during this process recommend ensuring that you have the laundry and other household chores caught up, including meal planning and prepping so that your mind can remain exclusively focused on the task at hand. There will be accidents- make sure you're not the cause of them because you were distracted taking care of some household chore!

The Potty Training in A Weekend method has gained steadily in popularity over the course of the last decade, particularly in Western countries, with varying degrees of difference in each guide. The guide provided in this book is set up in such a way that you can learn about the many variances to this methodology and choose to

adopt what you believe will work best for you and your little one. Just as every child is uniquely individual, so too is the home setup and the pattern of each individual household. View the guide here as a buffet of sorts: choose what you like and leave the rest.

Your results will vary because every child is an individual, but Potty Training in A Weekend method, when approached in a focused and mindful manner on the part of the parent and/or caregiver, is guaranteed to provide a bedrock foundation for your child's potty training prowess. Your goal should not be a 100% accident-free, potty using a child at the end of this weekend, but rather a child who is well on their way to becoming one.

Now that you have done the setup work to prime both yourself and your child to have the best mindset going into this process, you are ready to begin to delve into the step by step guide of potty training in a weekend.

Chapter 2: Potty Training in A Weekend

Day 1: Welcome to the Big Day!

Wake up and get yourself set up immediately with timer reminders before you even wake your child up for the day. Most people choose to use their smartphone for this, but if you do not have a smartphone, then any clock, watch or another electronic device that has a timer and alarm capability will do! It is best if it is a timer that is portable and you can move around with you as you move around your home, but if you are using a stationary alarm such as a microwave or stovetop, then just be aware of keeping the volume down on other electronics and outside noise throughout the day so you can hear the alarm.

The alarm will cue you to each and every time that you will need to take your child to sit on the potty. This should be approached as an exciting, fun thing for the first day. Every time the alarm sounds, react as if you are thrilled to be hearing it. Your child will catch on to this and be happy to hear it, too.

Your first alarm needs to be set for exactly 15 minutes after your child gets set up for the day, so set that up

as you go in to get your child out of bed. Building on what you began the day before, get your child out of bed in a fun and playful manner, reminding them of the exciting day you two have planned!

Keep your language here simple and direct so as not to confuse your child too much on what the day will contain. A sample script might sound something like this: "Today you get to start using the big kid potty just like <insert meaningful model here>! You get to wear big kid underwear and when you go big kid potty today, you'll get to pick a prize out of the treasure box! Let's take off this soggy diaper and pick out some big kid underwear!"

A lot of parents make a big production out of tossing this "last wet diaper" into the trash with their child and some even have the child toss it out and say something along the lines of "bye-bye diapers! I'm a big kid now!"

Let your child pick out their own underwear to wear and be sure that you comment on how fun it is to have underwear with their favorite character, pattern, or print on it. You can comment on the softness of the

material or the colors found on it. At some point during putting the underwear on, remind your child that underwear is not a diaper and that it is not meant to be peed or pooped in. Be sure to include something along the lines of, "do you feel like such a big kid with your big kid underwear on?"

Regarding the type of clothing your child should wear during this intensive potty training weekend, the only real requirement is that it needs to be something that your child can easily remove to sit on the potty. Many parents choose to just use an underwear and t-shirt combo, but anything that slides down and then back up easily will work. You don't want anything complicated that requires buttoning, zipping, or even Velcro because you don't want there to be any additional steps that your child will need to take to sit on the potty. You want to encourage as much independent movement as you can for your child around the potty. You want to help foster any associations between feeling capable and in control and use of the potty that you can.

Once you have gotten your child into their big kid underwear, it is time to begin the potty training process in earnest! Going into breakfast mode, allow your child to help you pick out what they would like for breakfast

and announce to them they get to have a special drink since it is the morning, they begin their potty training process. Give them one of their favorite beverages that you have picked out from the store and encourage them to drink up. Let them know that they are going to fill their belly up with their special drink and then be able to go sit on the big-kid potty. Once your child begins to drink, set the alarm for 15 minutes. This will be the first time you put your child on the potty, and hopefully, the sugary drink will have done the trick. Let your child know that when the alarm goes off, they will be able to go in and sit on the big kid potty!

Once the first fifteen-minute alarm sounds, this will be your time to really play up the event. React to the alarm as if it is the most exciting thing you have ever heard. Lead your child into the restroom (or depending on their excitement level, they can lead you!) and narrate the process as you go. "Alright! Here we go, off to your big kid potty. I'm so excited for you! This is great. Here we are, to the bathroom. Okay, can you pull your big kid underwear down, *all by yourself*? Awesome! Okay, now you can climb up to sit on your potty. Okay! Now let's check-in, see if there's any pee-pee in there that you

can put in the potty! <Show your child how to gently poke and put pressure on their lower abdomen, above their bladder> Do you feel some pee-pee in there? Let's see if you can put it in the potty!!!"

The cycle of drinking a beverage and then heading to the restroom will be repeated throughout this first day, but one of the most important aspects of this ritual will be in the narrative that you provide during this process. You want to continue to provide the child with the physical cues of where they will be feeling the pressure of their bladder, so they will make the association between the sensations of a full bladder and going to sit on the toilet.

For this first day, you will react with a celebration during every single visit to the potty. You want your child to experience a positive reinforcement of the association that going to the potty equals fun and happiness. It is not necessary that your child actually uses the potty chair, today you are celebrating just making the trip! You will celebrate each and every time they sit.

Allow your child two to three minutes to sit each time. During this time, stay with them. You can read a book about using the potty, listen to or sing a song about

using the potty, or watch one of the episodes about potty training available on various forms of media. Again, you are working to train your child to associate the sensations of a full bladder and pressure in their abdomen with the experience of sitting on the potty. Remember that you are building these connections from the ground up because they have never had to build them before! They have to move from mindless and passive elimination to conscious and mindful recognition and decision-making.

Again, this first day your child will get to pick a new treat from the treasure box each and every time they sit on the potty, regardless of if they go to the bathroom in the toilet or not. This first day is only for creating positive associations and teaching both toileting habits and how to be aware of their bodily sensations.

An Important Note About Accidents

Accidents will happen over the course of this weekend, especially on the first day. Do not be discouraged! Treat each accident as a neutral incident and keep your emotions level. Do not react as if it is a disappointment or a failure of any kind. A sample script for this scenario might be, "Ooops, it looks like you didn't make it to the

big kid potty. Let's go take this wet/dirty underwear over here and get all cleaned up. Next time, we will try to make it to the potty in time!"

Keep your narrative around potty accidents neutral and matter of fact. This is going to be a normal and natural part of the process and your child will be learning that when they go to the bathroom in their big kid underwear, it is a different sensation than when they went to the bathroom in their absorbent diaper.

Your child is making lots of new connections this weekend, one connection that they do NOT need to make is one of shame, disappointment, and disgust surrounding the toilet learning process. Keep your reactions neutral and matter of fact and they will adopt that same reaction.

In order to minimize your own stress and anxiety over accidents and the potential mess that can be made on furniture, some parents choose to either keep all activities for the day on the floor with a towel beneath the play space. Some parents even invest in some of the puppy pads that are available for dogs during crate training! These can even be put on furniture with regular bath towels over the top of them for both the

added protection of your furniture against accidents and also for the extra comfort for your child! Be sure to do the same for the child's spot at the dining room table, as well. Mealtimes can sometimes be an extra tricky time for new potty learners to navigate paying attention to their bodily sensations and signals while enjoying their meals!

Day one will proceed with the fifteen-minute intervals to sit on the toilet, keeping it an experience that the child wants to have with reading, singing, or media watching every time they sit on the toilet. Many catchy little jingles have been created surrounding potty use and they are helpful because children love catchy, rhyming, sing-songs phrases to begin with, and delivering helpful potty information is a way of reinforcing the potty experience for them. If you don't want to use one that has already been made, make up one for your family that you know your child will enjoy!

During the course of this first day, any time your child does actually pee or poop in the toilet, be sure to make a giant fuss over this! You want your child to feel proud and accomplished and to always reinforce that experience of elimination on the toilet with celebration and acknowledgment.

Going to bed that evening, be sure to tell your little one how very proud of them that you are, even if they didn't pee or poop in the potty a single time. Explain to them that because they will be asleep and unable to tell when they need to go potty, you will be putting special training pants on them (NOT their regular diapers, but something absorbent like a pull up) but will begin their awesome work on the potty again in the morning. This training takes a lot out of children, so be prepared for your kid to sleep like a log!

A Quick Note About Nighttime Potty Training

After a long day of visiting the restroom every fifteen minutes, you and your child will be exhausted! It can be tempting to introduce nighttime training at the same time but do be aware that this is not really something that can be trained but rather just something that a child outgrows and develops into. If your child often wakes up from their naps and their nightly sleep stretches dry, then nighttime training and trials with underwear have a great shot at success! However, it is very rare for a child to be dry during naps and nighttime sleep stretches but unable to control their bladder during the day. Typically, bladder awareness and potty training come before nighttime dryness.

By the age of six, approximately 85% of children will be able to stay dry, but children can continue to have nighttime accidents on occasion up until the age of 12 without it being considered an area of concern. Parents and caregivers know their children best and will be able to determine if nighttime toilet training should begin at the same time.

If you do choose to go this route, you will essentially continue the interval training as you do during the day, only with longer lengths in between. Instead of every fifteen minutes, you will set your alarm for every three hours and will pick up your child (because they will be half-asleep!) and carry them in to sit on the toilet. Some parents use audio cues to help their children use the restroom in the middle of the night by turning on a nearby faucet. Once the child has gone to the potty, return them to their bed.

In order to decrease some of the time spent dealing with nighttime accidents, it will be important to use a waterproof mattress protector underneath the regular sheets. Some parents even choose to do additional layers of waterproof mattress protectors and sheets so that way when an accident occurs, the wet layers of sheets can be easily stripped away and there will be a

dry layer already on the bed below. This can decrease nighttime sleep disruptions during the training process but do be aware that most nighttime potty training will be full of accidents if the child is not already mostly dry throughout the night. Again, this isn't really a training opportunity because nighttime bladder control has more to do with hormone production levels and those are produced on different timetables and have nothing to do with training.

Onward to Day Two!

Day two is much like day one, with one important difference. You will explain to your child that today, they will only be able to pick a treat out of the treasure box if they actually pee or poop in the potty. Do NOT mention accidents and be very careful about how you frame this information. You don't want your child to feel like they are being punished for having accidents, you want the emphasis to be on the reward for making it to the toilet!

Keep your spirits up and don't let up! This three-day potty training process is a *process*, not an event!

Day Three, Finally!

Day three is the day where big changes can often be seen. Explain to your child that today, you will be focusing on paying attention to your body and checking in. You will adjust your timer to half-hour increments, and rather than immediately traveling to the toilet to sit, you will instead encourage the "check-in."

"Let's stop and see if we need to go potty! <cue the gentle poking of the lower abdomen> Is there pee or poop in there that needs to come out? Should we go to try?" If it has been over an hour and your child still says they do not need the toilet and they have remained dry, encourage more drinking of fluids. Today is the day to really let your child figure out what these bodily sensations mean!

Chances are, your child is beginning to really connect the dots between what the feelings in their body mean and what they need to do about it. Day three is the day for them to really practice taking charge of this. You will still be checking in every half hour- and encouraging fluids- but you need to let them work out some of the cause and effect here, too.

Even if your child makes it to the toilet 100% on day 3, this does not mean that there will not be accidents moving forward! Small children are easily distracted and will still require some cueing and reminding the adults in their life. This is normal!

Read on for the next chapter if you find you have a Potty Training Outlier!

Chapter 3: Potty Training Outliers

Some children will potty train earlier than their peers and some will potty train later. This is just a normal part of this developmental process! If you have a child that has potty trained earlier than two, then you still may have some potty work coming in the future.

Potty training regression is when a child who was fully potty trained for a significant period of time begins having accidents consistently. If this is the case, you need to look at potential reasons why such as if there is an emotional or traumatic event occurring that needs addressed (toilet accidents are often present during times of abuse) or if extra support is needed day to day. Consult with your medical professional to rule out medical reasons such as a urinary tract infection or constipation.

For children who are beyond the age of four and still not interested in the potty or successful after an extended period of consistent potty training efforts, then this is also a scenario in which you might want to check in with a medical professional to see if there are any health issues at play that are causing the delay.

There are children who will potty train early and those that will potty train much later, but outliers exist on both ends and are typically not a cause for concern. Children who are not successful with potty training programs between the ages of two and four can spontaneously train themselves seemingly overnight when they decide that they are ready. Again, there is very little that children are able to have complete control over in their lives and the toileting process can be one of those things that children for reasons that adults may not understand. This does not mean your child is being manipulative or trying to be difficult; it means that they are trying to meet their own needs in the best way they know-how and support during this time means more emotional support than physical force.

Again, always speak to your child's doctor if you have any questions at all about health or well-being.

Bonus Chapter: Tips for Dads, From Dads

The relationship that a child has with their father is very unique and these are some tips and tricks that dads have shared with us:

"My little guy loves to do target practice in the toilet. I set him up with a few cheerios in the toilet and tell him to hit them as many times as he can and he is getting very good aim now!"

"My daughter loves to "show me how" so I like to pretend that I forgot how she uses the potty and she will walk me back to "show me how" and even sportscast the entire process!"

"I was worried about potty training and being away from home, but it's worked out really well so far. My son is really interested in all public restrooms, so anytime we end up at a store or restaurant, he immediately "has to go potty" which just means he wants to go see their restroom. It's working out though, not a single accident outside of the house!"

"Don't tell mom, but I still use Skittles. For pee on the potty, she gets two and for poop, she gets three. She never has an accident when I'm around."

"I let my daughter pick out a special foaming soap that she only gets to use after she's used the potty. It's sparkly blue and purple foam, so she makes sure that she makes it to the toilet so she can use some of her fancy "unicorn" soap!"

"I let my son pee in our backyard by our maple tree. We have a privacy fence so no one can see anything, and he LOVES it. I'm not sure what we will do in the winter, though…"

A lot of these dads have created playful ways to make the potty experience fun! Use your imagination to think of ways to do the same with your little one. Find ways to make this process tailored to you and your child and the this you like best.

Conclusion

Thank you for making it through to the end of **Potty Training in A Weekend:** *The Step-By-Step Guide to Potty Train Your Little Toddler in Less Than 3 Days. Perfect for Little Boys and Girls. Bonus Chapter with Tip for Careless Dads Included*, let's hope it was informative and able to provide you with all of the tools you need to achieve your goals in potty training your child.

Remember, potty training is a process and not an event. The three-day potty training method is intended to give your child a strong baseline knowledge of how to pay attention to and interpret the signals of their body and use the toilet properly. This doesn't mean that children will not have accidents as they go about their days, because children are easily distractible and after the fun of the three-day potty training method, going to sit on the potty won't seem quite as exciting as it did when they had a cheerleader on standby!

Continue to provide support for your child on their potty training journey and repeat the process as many times as you feel you need to. Remember that the potty training process requires a lot of your child: it is as

much a cognitive process as it is a physical one. Be sure to tell your child each and every night that they are doing a great job in learning how to use the big kid potty and that you are proud of all their hard work. Children that feel supported for their efforts, even when their efforts don't yield perfect results, will be far more likely to persist with determination than a child that is given the signals that because they did not do something perfectly that they have failed.

If you have been consistently potty training for an extended period of time with no results, consult with your child's doctor to rule out any possible medical issues. If none are present, then consider pausing the potty training process and revisiting it later. Keep your child in the loop of what is happening with as neutral language as you can. A sample script might sound like, "It seems like maybe you aren't quite ready to begin the big kid potty yet. We will try again in one month, okay?" It isn't a failure, just a standard part of the process involved in this major developmental leap! Kids that seem resistant at first may just need a little while longer to fully understand and grow comfortable with the process.

Besides, you can always be rest assured that everyone learns how to use the potty eventually. You will not be sending your child off to college in diapers, guaranteed! Just as some kids walk later than others, some will potty train later, too. The day will come, believe it or not, you might even miss the days when your little one was in diapers.

Finally, if you found this book useful in any way, a review on Amazon is always appreciated!

Potty Training for Newborn Superheroes

Say "Bye Bye" to Diapers in 72 Hours. The Perfect Guide for Busy Parents That Love Their Baby Genius.

By

MISSY RHYMES

Download the Audio Book Version of This Book for FREE

If you love listening to audio books on-the-go, I have great news for you. You can download the audio book version of this book for FREE just by signing up for a FREE 30-day audible trial! See below for more details!

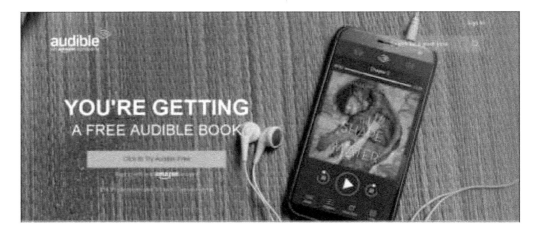

Audible Trial Benefits

As an audible customer, you will receive the below benefits with your 30-day free trial:

- FREE audible book copy of this book
- After the trial, you will get 1 credit each month to use on any audiobook
- Your credits automatically roll over to the next month if you don't use them
- Choose from Audible's 200,000 + titles
- Listen anywhere with the Audible app across multiple devices
- Make easy, no-hassle exchanges of any audiobook you don't love
- Keep your audiobooks forever, even if you cancel your membership
- And much more

Click the links below to get started!

For Audible US

For Audible UK

For Audible FR

For Audible DE

Table of Contents

Introduction

Parents play a key role in toilet training. Parents need to provide their child with direction, motivation, and reinforcement. They need to set aside time for and have patience with the toilet training process. Parents can encourage their child to be independent and allow their child to master each step at his or her own pace. WHEN TO BEGIN TOILET TRAINING YOUR CHILD There is no right age to toilet train a child the approximate time is between 15 months to 30 months.

Readiness to begin toilet training depends on the individual child. In general, starting before age 2 (24months) is not recommended. The readiness skills and physical development your child needs occur between age 18 months and 2.5 years.

Potty training might seem like a daunting task, but if your child is truly ready, there's not much to worry about. "Life goes on and one day your child will just do it," says Lisa Asta, M.D., a clinical professor of pediatrics at University of California, San Francisco, and spokesperson for the American Academy of Pediatrics. "When kids want to go on the potty, they will go on the

potty. Sometimes that happens at 18 months, sometimes it doesn't happen until close to age 4, but no healthy child will go into kindergarten in diapers." So don't stress — your child will ultimately get on the potty and do his thing, but you can help guide the process along. If you're ready to make diapers a thing of the past in your house, experts recommend following these seven easy steps.

Your child will show cues that he or she is developmentally ready. Signs of readiness include the fol-lowing:

• Your child can imitate your behavior.

• Your child begins to put things where they belong.

• Your child can demonstrate independence by saying "no."

• Your child can express interest in toilet training (e g, following you to the bathroom).

• Your child can walk and is ready to sit down.

• Your child can indicate first when he is "going"(urinating or defecating) and then when he needs to "go."

• Your child is able to pull clothes up and down (on and off).

Each child has his or her own style of behavior, which is called temperament. In planning your approach to toilet training, it is important to consider your child's temperament.

• Consider your child's moods and the time of day your child is most approachable.

Plan your approach based on when your child is most cooperative.

• If your child is generally shy and withdrawn, he or she may need additional support and encouragement.

• Work with your child's attention span.

Plan for distractions that will keep him or her comfortable on the potty chair. All this and many more on how to get your kid on potty will be explain in this ebook.

Chapter 1 What is potty training?

Potty training is teaching your child to recognize their body signals for urinating and having a bowel movement. It also means teaching your child to use a potty chair or toilet correctly and at the appropriate times.

1.1 When should toilet training start?

Potty training should start when your child shows signs that he or she is ready. There is no right age to begin. If you try to toilet train before your child is ready, it can be a battle for both you and your child. The ability to control bowel and bladder muscles comes with proper growth and development.

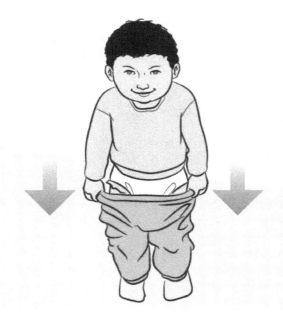

Children develop at different rates. A child younger than 12 months has no control over bladder or bowel movements. There is very little control between 12 to 18 months. Most children don't have bowel and bladder control until 24 to 30 months. The average age of toilet training is 27 months.

If you think your child is showing signs of being ready for toilet training, the first step is to decide whether you want to train using a potty or the toilet.

There are some advantages to using a potty – it's mobile and it's familiar, and some children find it less scary than a toilet. Try to find out your child's preference and go with that. Some parents encourage their child to use both the toilet and potty.

Second, make sure you have all the right equipment. For example, if your child is using the toilet you'll need a step for your child to stand on. You'll also need a smaller seat that fits securely inside the existing toilet seat, because some children get uneasy about falling in.

Third, it's best to plan toilet training for a time when you don't have any big changes coming up in your family life. Changes might include going on holiday, starting day care, having a new baby or moving house. It can be

a good idea to plan toilet training for well before or after these changes.

Also, toilet training might go better if you and your child have a regular daily routine. This way, the new activity of using the toilet or potty can be slotted into your normal routine

1.2 General Knowledge of potty for children

You may (happily) have noticed that you're changing fewer diapers lately and your little one is usually staying dry during nap time. These, along with other signs, indicate that it's time to dive into the world of potty training. The key to potty training success is patience and an awareness that all tots reach this ever important milestone at their own pace. Different strategies work with different children, but these tips generally get the job done.

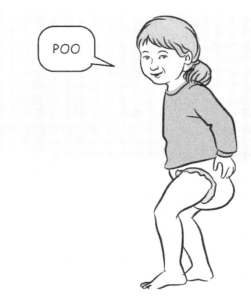

Since kids typically start potty training between 18 and 30 months, start talking about potty training occasionally around your child's first birthday to pique interest. Keep a few children's books about potty training lying around your house to read along with your child. And bring up the subject of the potty in conversation; saying things like, "I wonder if Elmo [or your child's favorite stuffed animal] needs to go potty" or "I have to go pee-pee. I'm headed to the potty." The idea is to raise awareness about going potty and make your child comfortable with the overall concept before he's ready to potty train.

If your child is staying dry for at least two hours during the day and is dry after naps, this could mean she's

ready to give the potty a shot. Before you head to the bathroom, know that she can follow simple instructions, like a request to walk to the bathroom, sit down, and remove her clothes. Also make sure she's interested in wearing big girl underwear. Then consider if she's aware when she's wet: If she cries, fusses, or shows other signs of obvious discomfort when her diaper is soiled and indicates through facial expression, posture, or language that it's time to use the toilet, then she's ready to start the process.

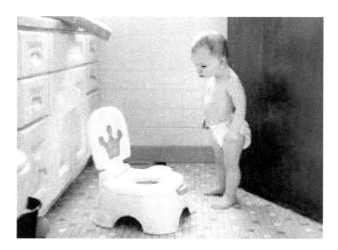

Some children are afraid of falling in the toilet or just hearing it flush, If your child is comfortable in the bathroom, try a potty seat that goes on top of your toilet to reduce the size of the bowl's opening. If not, you can buy a stand-alone potty chair and put it in the playroom or child's bedroom, where he'll become comfortable with

its presence over time. When he's ready to give it a try,

experts suggest you move it into the bathroom for repeated use, so you don't have to retrain your child down the road to transition from going potty in other rooms. Also get a stepstool—if he's using a potty seat, he'll need it to reach the toilet and also to give his feet support while he's pooping. "People can't empty their bowels and bladders completely unless their feet are pressing down on the floor.

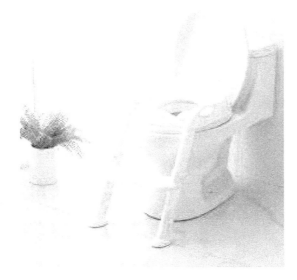

Even if your child seems ready, experts say to avoid potty training during transitional or stressful times. If you're moving, taking a vacation, adding a new baby to the family, or going through a divorce, postpone the potty training until about a month after the transitional time. Children trying to learn this new skill will do best if

they're relaxed and on a regular routine. You might prefer to get potty training over with as soon as

possible—maybe you're curious about the 3-day potty training trend. That's fine but do not always believe it, experts because you might find it frustrating not. "I often see parents who boast that they trained their 2-year-old in a weekend, and then say that the child has accidents four times a day, This is not the same as being potty trained. When kids are truly ready, they often will just start going on the potty on their own."

When you do decide it's time to start potty training, you'll want your child to go to the bathroom independently, day or night, so make sure she has transitioned out of

the crib and into a big-kid bed. "Kids need access to a potty 24/7 if they're potty training so they can reach it on their own when they need it. Keep a well-lit path to the bathroom so your child feels safe and comfortable walking there during the night. Of course, if you think you're child isn't ready for a big-kid bed (or, let's face it, if you're not ready), there's no harm in keeping her in diapers at night for a while longer. Talk to your child's doctor about the best time to potty train your child; the

answer will range greatly by child, though most kids should be out of diapers during the day by age 3. When you're ready to start training, let your child sit on the potty fully clothed when you are in the bathroom to get a feel for the seat. Then create a schedule: "The key is having times throughout the day where you ritualize using the potty so it becomes more of a habit," Dr. Swanson says. You might want to have him sit on the potty every two hours, whether he has to go or not, including first thing in the morning, before you leave the house, and before naps and bedtime. Tell him to remove his shorts or pants first, his underwear (or, if you're using them, training pants) next, and to sit on the toilet for a few minutes (allot more time, if you think he has to poop). Read him a book or play a game, like 20 Questions, to make the time pass in a fun way. Then, whether or not he actually goes potty, instruct him to flush and wash his hands. Of course, always praise him for trying.

It's not uncommon for a child who has been successfully using the potty for a few days to say he wants to go back to diapers. To avoid a power struggle or a situation where your child actually starts a pattern of withholding

bowel movements, which can lead to constipation, you might agree to a brief break. But try to build in a plan to resume by asking your child, "Would you like to wear underwear right when you get up or wait until after lunch?"

When you're potty training, accidents are part of the process; some kids still have accidents through age 5 or 6, and many don't stay dry at night until that age (or even later). Never punish your child for wetting or soiling his pants; he's just learning and can't help it. In fact, doing so might only make your little one scared of using the potty, and that, in turn, will delay the whole process even further. Instead, when your child uses the potty successfully, offer gentle praise and a small reward. You might want to use a sticker chart—your child receives a sticker every time he goes potty; after he's earned, say, three stickers, he gets a small prize. "However, don't go nuts!" Dr. Goldstein says. "A lot of toddlers will react to excessive praise as they react to punishment—by getting scared and avoiding doing the thing that they were excessively praised or punished for." In other words, stick with stickers, a trip to the local park, or even a surprise cup of hot cocoa—no need

to go on a shopping spree to Toys 'R' Us. Less tangible rewards, like finally living up to the promise of "being a

big kid" are enough for some kids. Remind your child about the benefits of "being a big kid," like if he wore underwear, he would never have to stop playing in order to get his diaper changed.So this should result to setting children up with good hygiene habits that will last a lifetime, washing hands should be a routine from Day 1, along with flushing and wiping, regardless of whether your child actually went in the potty. The Centers for Disease Control and Prevention recommends wetting hands with cool or warm running water, lathering up with soap, and scrubbing for at least 20 seconds. Make hand washing fun by buying colorful kid-friendly soaps, and make it last long enough by singing a favorite song, like "Happy Birthday to You" or the "ABC Song," so the bubbles work their germ-fighting magic. Yes, toilet training can be stressful—for the parents, that is! But if you follow your child's lead, it won't be stressful for him.

1.3 Dealing with the emotions

In this step-by-step guide, we are going to take you through some really in-depth training and information that my I have put together over the years on potty training. Additionally, When it comes to potty training, most parents and most people think it begins with the child. The reality is that potty training is begins with you, the parent or the grandparent, the relative or the daycare worker.

When we get testimonials from our clients and they say, "Thank you, thank you, thank you," I always like to say, "No, thank you. You are the one that did the hard work, so you are the one that deserves the congratulations." With that being said, we are going to start with you, the parent, or you, the person who is going to be doing the training.

You must be prepared and know that this is going to be a trying time, for some parents more than others. This can be a very stressful time because it tends to be a very stressful situation. What I want to make sure you understand is that nothing that is going on with your child with respect to potty training is your fault.

You have not done anything wrong. It may be as simple as the information you have received (or lack thereof). As an adult, what you know is that kids are not born knowing what to do and we are not born knowing how to be parents. Potty training, like many other lessons is something that is learned and you've taken the right steps in trying to acquire that information. So, the first step is to prepare yourself mentally for this project. Remember that your child has spent two or three years going to the bathroom in his or her diaper.

Now, you are going to ask them to do something that is completely out of the norm and, essentially erasing two or three years of habit. Saying that this is going to be a challenge may be an understatement as some children may battle and butt heads with you.

But being mentally prepared will help you in coping with the challenge itself. How do you get prepared? First, take your time, and get relaxed. Do whatever it takes to help you get into a relaxed state of mind. Its better if you can start the potty training process when have had a good amount of sleep. Being tired and trying to potty train makes it just that much more difficult.

You will also want to make sure your child is rested as

well. This is just as stressful for them and being cranky while learning a new technique is not a good combination. Also, practice counting to 10 and then counting backwards from 10. This is a practice that you will find calms you down during periods of frustration in the process. In addition to being relaxed, you will need

to ensure that you have a good support system. Talk with your husband or your wife or friends, and make sure that everyone is on board with what you are going to do so you are all heading in the same direction and can be a sounding board for each other.

This is critical because if there isn't a support system, the person doing the potty training will have a more difficult time and experience feelings of their own relating to the responsibility, frustration, and in some cases, failure (at least in the short run). If you are able to start this process on a weekend, it is highly suggested because you won't have the stress of work and you can have the dedicated focus needed to get this done right the first time. This can be applied to any period of time when you can get yourself a good three days to focus and concentrate.

1.4 Using motivation for the training

A lot of products out there will tell you that to motivate your child, you need to go to the store and pick up a toy or something like that. And while that's good, I want to give you something even better when it comes to motivation. Here's the problem with giving them toys or

saying, "I'm taking your toys away," and actually taking the toy away and hiding it so that they don't see it. When children are between the ages of 2 and 5, out of sight, out of mind, the average attention span at that age is about 7 minutes. So, if you take the toy away it only takes 7 minutes before they never even realized they had a toy in the first place. So, that motivation does not go very far. What I like to do is instead is use fear of loss versus fear of gain. Now, let me explain the difference to you between fear of loss and fear of gain. Most people even as adults think about it today. We work harder to prevent ourselves from losing things than we do to gain things. Fear of loss is a bigger motivator than fear of gain. So if you are saying, "If you behave, you will get..." or, "If you use the potty, you will get..." Although it can be a good thing for motivation, I think you can get a better response by saying, "If you don't

use the potty, you will lose this." In other words, if they don't use the potty, they're going to lose something.

Let me give you an example of one of the motivations we used to use with my youngest son. We had to "outsmart the fox" as I call it. I used to have to say something like, "Lorenzo, do you want to go to

McDonald's?" And he'd say, "Yes, let's go toMcDonald's." So, then I would say, "Okay, great. Go get your coat. Go get your shoes. Let's go to McDonalds." He'd go get his stuff and we'd open the front door and get ready to walk out. And then I would say, "Oh, you know what Lorenzo, let's use the bathroom before we go because you don't want to have an accident at Ronald McDonald's house." So, what did I do it at that point? Using a fear of loss, I defuse the potty. At that point, losing McDonalds was way more important to him than the toilet. So, he went without any issues at all. Now, granted, going to McDonald's means you have to spend money, but there are other ways that you can use the same methodology inside the house. For example, you can use their favorite cookie or their favorite snack.

Let's say they like pudding. You might say, "Hey Lorenzo, do you want some pudding?" And the answer of

course is going to be, "Yes." You then take the pudding, you put it on the table, you put the spoon in the bowl, you actually let them grab the spoon, get ready to take a bite and you say, "Wait a second, wait a second. Before you take that bite, let's go use the potty." At this point, the pudding and the reward are so real to the child that the potty is nothing. They'll use the potty just so they can come back and get that reward. You can do this with the toys as well.You can also do it with television. If it is a television program that they really like, then I would wait until the show is getting ready to start and I'd say, "Hey, let's go use the bathroom before we have an accident watching the show." If they said, "Oh the show is starting. I don't want to use the bathroom." Then, your answer is, "Well, we better go quickly if you want to see that show. Until we use the bathroom the show is not going to be on." Then, you can literally turn the television off. So, that is the way to motivate getting to the results. You don't want to use the same old, "I'm taking the toys away." You hide the toys and they don't see the toys for months, and to them, they never existed in the first place.

1.5 How will I know my toddler is ready to be potty trained?

If your little one isn't developmentally ready for potty training, even the best toilet tactics will fall short. Wait for these surefire signs that your tot is set to get started: You're changing fewer diapers. Until they're around 20 months old, toddlers still pee frequently, but once they can stay dry for an hour or two, it's a sign that they're developing bladder control and are becoming physically ready for potty training.

Bowel movements become more regular. This makes it easier to pull out the potty in a pinch when it's time. Your little one is more vocal about going to the bathroom. When your child starts to broadcast peeing and pooping by verbalizing or showing you through his facial expressions, potty training is on the horizon.

Your child notices (and doesn't like) dirty diapers. Your little one may suddenly decide she doesn't want to hang out in her dirty diapers because they're gross. Yay! Your child is turning her nose up at stinky diapers just like you do and is ready to use the potty instead. Kids are generally not ready to potty train before the age of 2, and some children may wait until 3 1/2. It's important to remember not to push your child before he's ready and to be patient. And remember that all kids are different. Your child is not developmentally lagging if he's far into his 3s before he gets the hang of potty training. Potty training success hinges on physical, developmental and behavioral milestones, not age. Many children show

signs of being ready for potty training between ages 18 and 24 months. However, others might not be ready until they're 3 years old. There's no rush. If you start too early, it might take longer to train your child.

1.6 Is your child ready? Ask yourself:

λ Can your child walk to and sit on a toilet?

λ Can your child pull down his or her pants and pull them up again?

λ Can your child stay dry for up to two hours?

λ Can your child understand and follow basic directions?

λ Can your child communicate when he or she needs to go?

λ Does your child seem interested in using the toilet or wearing "big-kid" underwear?

If you answered mostly yes, your child might be ready. If you answered mostly no, you might want to wait especially if your child is about to face a major change, such as a move or the arrival of a new sibling.

Your readiness is important, too. Let your child's motivation, instead of your eagerness, lead the process. Try not to equate potty training success or difficulty with your child's intelligence or stubbornness. Also, keep in

mind that accidents are inevitable and punishment has no role in the process. Plan toilet training for when you or a caregiver can devote the time and energy to be consistent on a daily basis for a few months.

1.7 How to know when its time for a child with special need

While parents often complain of difficulty potty training their children, for most families, potty training is a fairly easy experience. Even when there are problems or children show signs of potty training resistance, usually, they will eventually become potty trained.

1.8 Signs of Potty Training Readiness in Children With Special Needs

However, this is not always the case for children with developmental delays or disabilities, such as autism, Down syndrome, mental retardation, cerebral palsy, etc. Children with special needs can be more difficult to potty train. Most children show signs of physical readiness to begin using the toilet as toddlers, usually between 18 months and 3 years of age 1, but not all children have the intellectual and/or psychological readiness to be

potty trained at this age. It is more important to keep your child's developmental level, and not his chronological age in mind when you are considering starting potty training.

Signs of intellectual and psychological readiness includes being able to follow simple instructions and being cooperative, being uncomfortable with dirty diapers and wanting them to be changed, recognizing when he has a full bladder or needs to have a bowel movement, being able to tell you when he needs to urinate or have a bowel movement, asking to use the potty chair or asking to wear regular underwear.

Signs of physical readiness can include your being able to tell when your child is about to urinate or have a bowel movement by his facial expressions, posture or by what he says, staying dry for at least 2 hours at a time, and having regular bowel movements. It is also helpful if he can at least partially dress and undress himself.

1.9 Potty Training Challenges

Children with physical disabilities may also have problems with potty training that involves learning to get on the potty and getting undressed. A special potty chair and other adaptations may need to be made for these children.

Things to avoid when toilet training your child, and help prevent resistance, are beginning during a stressful time or period of change in the family (moving, new baby, etc.), pushing your child too fast, and punishing mistakes. Instead, you should treat accidents and mistakes lightly. Be sure to go at your child's pace and show strong encouragement and praise when he is successful.

Since an important sign of readiness and a motivator to begin potty training involves being uncomfortable in a

dirty diaper, if your child isn't bothered by a soiled or wet diaper, then you may need to change him into regular underwear or training pants during daytime training. Other children can continue to wear a diaper or pull-ups if they are bothered, and you know when they are dirty. Once you are ready to begin training, you can choose a potty chair. You can have your child decorate it with stickers and sit on it with his clothes on to watch TV, etc. to help him get used to it. Whenever your child shows signs of needing to urinate or have a bowel movement, you should take him to the potty chair and explain to him what you want him to do. Make a consistent routine of having him go to the potty, pull down his clothes, sit on the potty, and after he is finished, pulling up his clothes and washing his hands. At first, you should only keep him seated for a few minutes at a time, don't insist and be prepared to delay training if he shows resistance. Until he is going in the potty, you can try to empty his dirty diapers into his potty chair to help demonstrate what you want him to do.

1.10 Tips for Potty Training Children With Developmental Delays

An important part of potty training children with special needs is using the potty frequently. This usually includes scheduled toileting as outlined in the book Toilet Training Without Tears by Dr. Charles E. Schaefer. This "assures that your child has frequent opportunities to use the toilet." Sitting on the potty should occur "at least once or twice every hour" and after you first ask, "Do you have to go potty?" Even if he says no, unless he is totally resistant, it is a good idea to take him to the potty anyway. If this routine is too demanding on your child, then you can take him to the potty less frequently. It

can help to keep a chart or diary of when he regularly wets or soils himself so that you will know the best times to have him sit on the potty and maximize your chances that he has to go. He is also most likely to go after meals and snacks and that is a good time to take him to the potty. Frequent visits during the times that he is likely to use the potty and fewer visits to the potty at other times of the day is another good alternative. Other good techniques include modeling, where you allow your child to see family members or other children using the

toilet, and using observational remarks. 4 This involves narrating what is happening and asking questions while potty training, such as "Did you just sit on the potty?" or "Did you just poop in the potty?" Even after he begins to use the potty, it is normal to have accidents and for him to regress or relapse at times and refuse to use the potty. Being fully potty trained, with your child recognizing when he has to go to the potty, physically goes to the bathroom and pulls down his pants, urinates or has a bowel movement in the potty, and dresses himself, can take time, sometimes up to three to six months. Having accidents or occasionally refusing to use the potty is normal and not considered resistance.

Early on in the training, resistance should be treated by just discontinuing training for a few weeks or a month and then trying again. In addition to a lot of praise and encouragement when he uses or even just sits on the potty, material rewards can be a good motivator. This can include stickers that he can use to decorate his potty chair or a small toy, snack or treat. You can also consider using a reward chart and getting a special treat if he gets so many stickers on his chart.

You can also give treats or rewards for staying dry. It

can help to check to make sure he hasn't had an accident between visits to the potty. If he is dry, then getting very excited and offering praise, encouragement, and maybe even a reward, can help to reinforce his not having accidents.

1.11 How to Use Positive Practice for Accidents

Another useful technique is positive practice for accidents. Dr. Schaefer describes this as what you should do when your child has an accident and wets or soils himself.

This technique involves firmly telling your child what he has done, taking him to the potty where he can clean and change himself (although you will likely need to help) and then having him practice using the potty. Dr. Schaefer recommends going through the usual steps of using the potty at least five times, starting when "the child walks to the

toilet, lowers his pants, briefly sits on the toilet (3 to 5 seconds), stands up, raises his pants, washes his hands, and then returns to the place where the accident occurred."

Although you are trying to teach him the consequences of having an accident, this should not take the form of punishment.

1.12 When to Get Help for Special Needs Kids With Potty Training Difficulties

While it may take some time and require a lot of patience, many children with special needs can be potty trained by the age of 3 to 5 years. 3 If you continue to have problems or your child is very resistant, then consider getting professional help.

In addition to your pediatrician, you might get help from an occupational therapist, especially if your child has some motor delays causing the potty training difficulty, a child psychologist, especially if your child is simply resistant to potty training and a developmental pediatrician

1.13 When it's time to begin potty training:

Choose your words. Decide which words you're going to

use for your child's bodily fluids. Avoid negative words, such as dirty or stinky.

Prepare the equipment. Place a potty chair in the bathroom or, initially, wherever your child is spending most of his or her time. Encourage your child to sit on the potty chair in clothes to start out. Make sure your child's feet rest on the floor or a stool. Use simple, positive terms to talk about the toilet. You might dump the contents of a dirty diaper into the potty chair and toilet to show their purpose. Have your child flush the toilet. Schedule potty breaks. Have your child sit on the potty chair or toilet without a diaper for a few minutes at two-hour intervals, as well as first thing in the morning and right after naps. For boys, it's often best to master urination sitting down, and then move to standing up after bowel training is complete. Stay with your child and read a book together or play with a toy while he or she sits. Allow your child to get up if he or she wants. Even if your child simply sits there, offer praise for trying — and remind your child that he or she can try again later. Bring the potty chair with you when you're away from home with your child.

Get there

Fast! When you notice signs that your child might need to use the toilet such as squirming, squatting or holding the genital area respond quickly. Help your child become familiar with these signals, stop what he or she is doing, and head to the toilet. Praise your child for telling you when he or she has to go. Keep your child in loose, easy-to-remove clothing.

Explain hygiene. Teach girls to spread their legs and wipe carefully from front to back to prevent bringing germs from the rectum to the vagina or bladder. Make sure your child washes his or her hands afterward. Ditch the diapers. After a couple of weeks of successful potty breaks and remaining dry during the day, your child might be ready to trade diapers for training pants or underwear. Celebrate the transition. Let your child return to diapers if he or she is unable to remain dry. Consider using a sticker or star chart for positive reinforcement.

Chapter 2 Getting started with toilet training

The following tips may help you get started with potty training:

If there are siblings, ask them to let the younger child see you praising them for using the toilet.

It's best to use a potty chair on the floor rather than putting the child on the toilet for training. The potty chair is more secure for most children. Their feet reach the floor and there is no fear of falling off. If you decide to use a seat that goes over the toilet, use a footrest for your child's feet. Let your child play with the potty. They can sit on it with clothes on and later with diapers off. This way they can get used to it. Never strap your child to the potty chair. Children should be free to get off the potty when they want. Your child should not sit on the potty for more than 5 minutes. Sometimes children have a bowel movement just after the diaper is back on because the diaper feels normal. Don't get upset or punish your child. You can try taking the dirty diaper off and putting the bowel movement in the potty with your child watching you. This may help your child understand that you want the bowel movement in the potty.

If your child has a normal time for bowel movements (such as after a meal), take your child to the potty at that time of day. If your child acts a certain way when having a bowel movement (such as stooping, getting quiet, going to the corner), try taking your child to potty when he or she shows it is time.

If your child wants to sit on the potty, stay next to your child and talk or read a book. It's good to use words for what your child is doing (such as potty, pee, or poop). Then your child learns the words to tell you. Remember that other people will hear these words. Don't use words that will offend, confuse, or embarrass others or your child. Don't use words such as dirty, naughty, or stinky to describe bowel movements and urine. Use a simple, matter-of-fact tone.

If your child gets off the potty before urinating or passing a bowel movement, be calm. Don't scold. Try again later. If your child successfully uses the potty, give plenty of praise such as a smile, clap, or hug. Children learn from copying adults and other children. It may help if your child sits on the potty chair while you are using the toilet.

Children often follow parents into the bathroom. This

may be one time they are willing to use the potty. Start out by teaching boys to sit down for passing urine. At first, it is hard to control starting and stopping while standing. Boys will try to stand to urinate when they see other boys standing.

Some children learn by pretending to teach a doll to go potty. Get a doll that has a hole in its mouth and diaper area. Your child can feed and "teach" the doll to pull down its pants and use the potty. Make this teaching fun for your child.

Make going to the potty a part of your child's daily routine. Do this first thing in the morning, after meals and naps, and before going to bed.

2.1 After training is started

The following tips may help you once the training is started:

Once your child starts using the potty and can tell you they need to go, taking them to the potty at regular times or reminding them too many times to go to the potty is not necessary.

You may want to start using training pants. Wearing underpants is a sign of growing up, and most children

like being a "big girl or big boy." Wearing diapers once potty training has been started may be confusing for your child.

If your child has an accident while in training pants, don't punish. Be calm and clean up without making a fuss about it.

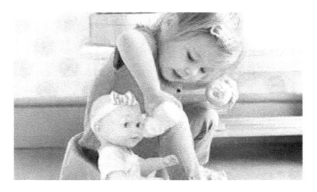

Keep praising or rewarding your child every step of the way. Do this for pulling down pants, for sitting on the potty, and for using the potty. If you show that you are pleased when your child urinates or has bowel movements in the potty, your child is more likely to use the potty next time. As children get older, they can learn to wipe themselves and wash hands after going to the bathroom. Girls should be taught to wipe from front to back so that germs from bowel movement are not wiped into the urinary area. Remember that every child is different and learns toilet training at his or her own

pace. If things are going poorly with toilet training, it's better to put diapers back on for a few weeks and try again later. In general, have a calm, unhurried approach to toilet training.

Most children have bowel control and daytime urine control by age 3 or 4. Soiling or daytime wetting after this age should be discussed with your child's healthcare provider.

Nighttime control usually comes much later than daytime control. Complete nighttime control may not happen until your child is 4 or 5 years old, or even older. If your child is age 5 or older and does not stay dry at night, you should discuss this with your child's healthcare provider.

Even when children are toilet trained, they may have some normal accidents (when excited or playing a lot), or setbacks due to illness or emotional situations. If accidents or setbacks happen, be patient. Examples of emotional situations include moving to a new house, a family illness or death, or a new baby in the house. In fact, if you know an emotional situation is going to be happening soon, don't start toilet training. Wait for a calmer time.

2.2 Potty Training Chairs

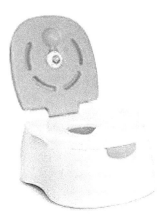

Many parents ask, "Do I need a potty training chair to be successful in potty training?" The answer to that question is "yes" and "no". For even our own kids, I used potty training chairs for two and no potty training chairs for our third child.

Now, he was an advanced child. He was doing things that the other kids never did so he never even wanted to use the potty chair. Even today as a 6-year-old in kindergarten, he doesn't like doing things that the other kindergarten kids like to do.

He calls them "babies." But I will tell you this: having a potty training chair does several things for your child. First of all, it gives them flexibility. When they have a potty training chair, more than likely it is mobile, which

means that it can be placed anywhere around the house including the TV room or the game room.

This increases the success rate of your child using the potty. The rationale? Well, as you might already know, if you're in any other room than the bathroom when you see kids doing a pee-pee dance or you realize that they've got to go, it's already too late. That pee or the bowel movement is almost on its way out the door.

But with a mobile potty chair, you can place it near their activities and in different rooms, so when the child feels the need to go, they don't have to rush all the way to the bathroom. They can simply get up and go in the vicinity of wherever they are.

Not only that, the act of running and holding for child that young is a very challenging thing. So trying to run to the bathroom from outside is almost asking for trouble. What you want to do instead is make sure that if you are going to use a potty chair, is that it's available and near. A potty chair is also great especially if you have a 2-story house and the bathroom is upstairs. You can then put the potty chair downstairs and cut out that climb. And the way potty chairs are designed today, they're colorful, they are cute and kids love them. It just

is a fun thing for them and they always get a sense of pride because it's their chair and nobody else's. What we used to do is put the potty chair in a laundry room because there was a door there. My son would be able to close the door so we couldn't see him and he would have his privacy.

2.3 Starting the process

There are three different times that you can start the training process.

Early — when the child is 2 or younger Middle — between the ages of 2 and 3, maybe 3 1/2 Later — between 3, 3 1/2 and older The optimal time for me is the age of 2.

And, I mean the day they turned 2 is when we normally like to start with potty training. With all the years that I have been in day care and all the children that I have

potty trained, I started every single one the day they turned 2. Even our own kids, we started them at the age of 2.

Now, starting at a later time is okay and that is the case with most parents. But I want to explain to you the

difference between starting at the age of 2 and starting later. The key difference in starting at the age of 2 is that the child hasn't developed all of their social skills yet and their ability to go out and have fun is limited.

At the age of 2 and somewhere between 2 and 3 is when they find their own voice. (You've heard of the terrible '2s'!?) They find their own voice and they find their own spirit and that's when they decide that they want to start doing their own thing. When you start earlier in the potty training process it is easier to get them to follow directions and it is just easier to get them to do what you want them to do versus them wanting to do what they want to do. Now, girls can start even earlier than 2. Usually girls can start about 3 or 4 months before their 2nd birthday. Girls, as we know, even later on in life, are a lot smarter than boys and men, and I will be the first to admit that.

The earliest we've seen was a little girl in my class that was only 15 months that was potty training and doing a fantastic job. But some kids can start as early as 18 or 19 months, including boys. So, potty training earlier is great because it gives you the ability to control the process versus them being in control. When you start at

that middle time frame, which is between 2 and 3 or 2 1/2 to 3 or later than that, what happens is that child goes more into the independent stage.

That's where they're able to start making to some of their decisions which happens to often include the word "no". And thus what happens as a parent is you're not only dealing with potty training but you're also dealing with behavior as the result of a child that is looking to find their self and their voice. Starting late doesn't mean you did anything wrong, and it doesn't mean that you're not going to potty train.; All it means is that it's going to be a little bit more challenging and a little bit more work. And that's okay but it just means that it's going to take a little bit more time to get the child potty trained.

Now, the other thing that you want to realize is the later you start, the more years of behavior modification you're trying to reverse and that can account for some of that difficulty. In other words, when you start the potty training at the age of 2, you only have 2 years of pooping in their diaper or potty in the diaper to reverse. Whereas the later you start, let's say at the age of 3, you've got 3, 3 1/2 years of pooping in their diaper or the potty behavior that you have to reverse. So, it's a

very big difference starting earlier than later because it's a lot more habit that has to be broken and a new habit learned.

To drive this point home, just think about how hard it is to change a behavior or a habit in yourself. If you think it's hard for yourself, think about a child that doesn't have the same cognitive ability that you have. Trying to get rid of that behavior as early as possible is better because it's less work for the child. We want to keep in mind how hard that child actually has to work to do this. The key also is that we're looking at doing this in just 3 days through consistency. So, reversing years of behavior in just 3 days is even that much more challenging the older they are.

2.4 Pre-potty training

Pre-potty training is getting the child ready for what is about to come if you really want to potty train him within 3 days, or what it is about to happen. In other words, you set a time when you're going to start potty training. It's now February and you want to start potty-training in September or something to that effect. Before

September comes around, there are things that you can

do that will make the potty training process not only easier for yourself, but also easier for the child.

The first thing you want to do is sit your child down and explain what is expected of them. Sitting down is an important component of this.

You want to sit next to them or across from them and in a very loving and caring tone, you want to say, "I am going to explain potty training to you." And you want to say, "Potty training is when you go the bathroom (tinkle, pee or poopy) in the potty." Now in terms of the words that you use, you want to be consistent. If you call it "tinkle" then you want to continue using the word "tinkle". If you call it "poopy", then continue using the word "poopy".

As a young child, too many words are going to confuse them, so staying consistent with your terminology will help you enforce the concept and they will know exactly what it means. You want to be strong and direct.

By that I mean using words like, "Mommy is going to have you potty trained, and here's what you have to do for Mommy...poopy, tinkle, etc." Or, "When you have to go potty, you have to let Mommy know, and you have to sit on the toilet and then you go potty". Then, you

physically walk them to the toilet and show them and say, "Here is where you go tinkle and poopy." This isn't being strict; it's being direct so that they know that you are in charge, and what is expected of them.

If you don't take it direct tone, kids are extremely smart. They can sense a lack of control and they might not follow your directions as well if you say, "Mommy would like" or, "It would be nice if you...""".

Take them to the bathroom and get them use to seeing you in the bathroom. Let them sit down on the toilet. Let them get used to having the toilet touch their skin as well. Many parents don't realize this, but many children have a fear of being on the toilet as opposed to just being hard to potty train. So this might help them get over that fear so when the potty training begins, you don't have to battle two things.

One thing is to start using less absorbent diapers. Today, the diapers are so absorbent the child doesn't even realize that they are wet. And most kids do not like the feeling of being wet. So when they have on a less absorbent diaper, it helps them realize the act of letting go and releasing 'number 1'. But the wet feeling also starts to psychologically or subconsciously say to them,

"When I get this feeling of letting go, I start to feel wet too, and I don't like that." You will also want to make sure that you change them frequently when they wet their diapers. This helps them get used to the feeling of being dry and staying dry. It also reinforces the feelings they have once they wet again. It is also highly encouraged that you actually consider taking your child out of diapers while they are awake a couple of months prior to the actual potty training process. So, during nap time, you will use diapers, but during their waking hours, you will want them in big boy and big girl underwear. You will also want to make sure that this whole pre-potty training process is a loving experience because you want it to subconsciously erase some of the other negative connotations and fears that your child may have. It's important that you understand pre potty training is not a necessary step. It gives you an advantage if you are starting the potty training process early, but if you are like most parents, then you might have missed the stage or the time when you could have pre-potty trained. You can still pre-potty train if you prefer, no matter at which stage you are, but it's

usually better if you can start as early as possible.

Knowing what we know and from our customers, however, most parents usually has missed this stage to the degree that they can get the most effectiveness out of it.

Chapter 3 Four stages of Potty training

In this section, I am going to teach you four stages to potty training. What you will notice and then appreciate is that these four stages can be applied to almost any other learned or practiced behavior which you are trying to alter or change.

3.1 The four stages of any behavior modification model include:

- Unconscious incompetence

- Conscious incompetence

- Conscious competence

- Unconscious competence

And now, I'll break these down to help you understand what they are and what you need to focus on during each one of these different stages.

Stage One: Unconscious Incompetence:

This is the "I do not know" stage, where your child's mind is thinking, "I do not know that going to the bathroom in my diaper is a wrong thing". In other words, the child has no idea that what they are doing is something they should not be doing. During stage one,

when they don't know the difference, this is when it becomes your responsibility to educate them and get them to understand what they are doing is not something they should be doing.

This is where you are teaching the child that they do not need to be going to the bathroom in their diaper.

Stage Two: Conscious Incompetence

At this stage, the child has reached an understanding where they know what they're doing is something they should not do, but have no idea how to correct it. During stage two you are taking it to that next level where you are reinforcing the positive behavior by showing them where they are supposed to go to the bathroom—in the potty. So, now you're teaching the child where to go, how to go, and what to do.

Stage Three: Conscious Incompetence

Here, the child knows what they are doing is something they shouldn't be doing, they know what to do about it, but they are also not that great at it. They have to think about it. That is because the process is now occurring on the conscious level. It is during stage three that the child starts to understand on their own and they start to show you the signs that they can do this on their own as well.

This is when you should be getting to the point of not having accidents anymore. Now, this is an area where most parents go wrong in that they get to stage three and they say, "My child is potty trained, there is nothing else that I have to do." In reality, this is where the real potty training begins. This is where you really want to be consistent to ensure they reach stage four and can consistently go to the potty by themselves. So, when you get to stage three, you have to make sure that you continue with consistency.

Stage Four: Unconscious Competence

And this is the fun stage. This is when the child gets to where they need to should know what they're doing and they don't have to think about it any longer. It is at stage four that your child can be officially considered 'potty trained.' Let's take a quick example to make sure the concept sinks in: If you are in stage three, you're not showing the child where to go potty anymore because they know where to go. What you're doing is being consistent with them going to the potty on a regular basis. During stage two you're not so much worried about consistency yet, you are more focused on helping them know where to go. Hopefully this description has given you a better understanding of how each stage develops and, better yet, what your actions need to be during each stage.

3.2 Potty Training as a young Mother

As a young mum who have no much experience about potty training; one of the best thing you can do to help your kid is to be a positive potty model. When you go to the bathroom, use it as an opportunity to talk your child through the process. Use words he or she can say, like pee, poop, and potty.

If you plan to start your child on a potty seat, put it in the bathroom so it becomes familiar. Make it a fun place your child wants to sit, with or without the diaper on. Have your child sit on the potty seat while you read or offer a toy.

Also, tune in to cues. Be aware of how your child behaves when he has to pee or poop. Look for a red face and listen for grunting sounds. Take notice of the time when he pees and poops during the day. Then establish a routine in which your child sits on the potty during those times, especially after meals or after drinking a lot of fluid. This helps set your child up for success.

And use plenty of praise, praise, and more praise. Is your child motivated by verbal encouragement? Stickers on a chart? Small toys or extra bedtime stories? Check in with what feels right for you and use it to reward positive potty choices. Your good attitude will come in handy, especially when "accidents" happen.

3.3 What Not to Do

Sitting on the potty should be a want-to, not a have-to. If your child isn't into it, don't force it.

Just when you think your child has nailed it, accidents happen. It's OK to be frustrated, but don't punish or shame your child -- it won't get you closer to your goal. Take a deep breath and focus on what you and your child can do better next time. Also, don't compare your son or daughter with other children. Some parents like to brag about how easy potty training went in their family. So if your neighbor says her kids potty trained themselves, smile and remember that the only right way is the one that works for you.

And if you a working mum, you juggle all your professional and personal responsibilities and, somehow, you make it look simple. Life is busy, though, and you've

got a huge task to add to the to-do list: learning how to potty-train.

Helping your little one switch from diapers to the bathroom is a tough job — regardless of whether you're a stay-at-home or working parent. Because you fall into the latter category, you have to plan the process more carefully, so you are present for the majority of the transition. As you prepare for life without diapers, here are some tips to keep in mind to make it simpler for you as you balance your professional schedule and potty-train schedule.

1. Choose the Right Time

Parenting books will probably suggest the perfect time to start potty-training, but no two children are the same. Some little ones start using the potty at as young as 24 months, but that's rare. In most cases, children begin between 24 and 36 months, and the entire process can take up to eight months to perfect after that.

Still, you should be more focused on starting the process when your child shows they are ready for it. For instance, some kids will start to show interest in their siblings' or classmates' potty behavior, which can help you ease them into using the toilet, too. Also, if your

child sleeps through nap time without wetting their diaper, they could be prepared to potty-train. To that end, staying dryer for longer also shows a little one has what it takes to wear big-kid underwear. Finally, your child might alert you when they must go, hide when they have to pee or poop, or tug at a dirty diaper.

Once you start seeing these cues, you should start thinking about beginning the process. There's no need to start too soon and put too much on your plate when you're already busy.

2. Invest in the Tools

Now that you know it's time to potty-train, you have to invest in the supplies you need to make it possible. For one thing, you'll need to pick up some underwear for your son or daughter. On a weekend or after-work trip to the store, bring your child along to help pick out their designs — they'll find it even more exciting to switch to underwear if they like the character or colors. Having the proper clothing and underwear, along with other potty-training supplies like extra bed sheets, flushable wipes, and soap you can keep your child comfortable and ready for anything.

However, mistakes happen! If they do make a mess,

teach them to not put anything other than toilet paper or flushable wipes in the toilet! By preventing the flushing of wipes and the use of too much paper, you will minimize the amount of plumbing-related issues you will experience. When clogs do occur, knowing how to effectively use a plunger and when to call in a plumber can also save you a lot of grief.

3. Work with Teachers or Nannies

You can kick off your potty-training extravaganza over the weekend but, by Monday, you'll have to go back to work. Rather than halting your progress and popping your child back into diapers, work with their nanny or preschool teacher so everyone's on the same page about the transition. Chances are, your childcare provider will be more than willing to stick to the routine you've started, as well as any rewards system you have in place. Think about it — it's beneficial for them not have to change diapers anymore, either. Make sure you pack plenty of dry clothes just in case, as accidents do happen. Then, once you pick up your child and go home, you can continue the training process yourself.

4. Reward Good Potty Habits

Experts have varying opinions on rewarding children for

their successful use of the potty. Some say it's a great way to boost their accountability, while others think the feeling of being clean and dry is reward enough. It's up to you whether or not you'll incentivize the process with treats, stickers or a potty-training chart.

No matter what, it's vital that you verbalize how proud you are of your child as they use the potty. Even if their teachers take the reins during the day, shower them with praise as soon as you pick them up and hear updates on the process. It can be frustrating if your child fusses about using the toilet or if they suffer from accidents, but you can't let them see or feel this from you. With a supportive parent helming the transition from diapers to potty, children are more likely to try.

Start and Succeed

Once you've pinpointed the right time to start, invested in the right gear and enlisted the help of your child's teachers, you're ready to potty-train. You'll be surprised how these simple steps can make it so much easier to get the job done, even while you're working. Cheer your child to the finish line both of you will be freer and happier sans diapers, which is the best benefit of all.

3.4 How to Potty Train a Child with Special Needs as a mum

If you have a child with special needs, then you know that you may not be able to rely on the "typical" signs of potty training readiness. Kristen Raney from Shifting Roots shares her experience with potty training her son.

Potty Training a Child on the Autism Spectrum First of all, don't read those stories about moms who potty train their children in three days!!! This will not work for our children and will cause you so much stress!! Remember through this process that you are a good mom doing the best you can for your child.

Most of the moms of autistic children I know were not able to potty train their children before four, many of them five, and some of them never. It just depends where your child falls on the Autism Spectrum and what their particular sensory issues are.

For context, our son would be considered to have Aspergers, but it's no longer a diagnosis and is now part of the Autism Spectrum. His body was ready to potty train around 2 1/2, but he had very intense fears about using the toilet. No bribe, game, song, or sticker chart in

the world could get him to use it. He also was terrified to pee or poo in pre-K, daycare, or anywhere in public. We started by getting him trained to pee on the potty, and he hit that milestone by 3 1/2. I don't remember how, because it was so stressful that I've erased that time from my mind. I think it involved making him pee in his diaper in the bathroom, and slowly transferring that idea to the potty. Once he got that, he had to ask for a diaper if he wanted to poo, and go in his diaper in the bathroom. To get him trained all the way, it took a 90 minute battle of wills where I told him he could poop on the potty or on the bathroom floor, it was entirely his choice. It was terrible. He chose the potty, glared at me like I was killing him. We bought him a Thomas train for the next three times he went on the potty, and a fourth one for keeping it up for a week. Yes, this sounds completely excessive and terrible, but he was 4 1/4 and we were at our wits end.

I hope your journey is much less stressful than ours, but know that you're not alone! Don't take any flack from someone with a neurotypical kid who gives you grief about not having your child trained by now. You've got this mama!

3.5 How to Potty Train a "Late" Bloomer

Here's the thing. Out of all of my mom friends, not one of our kiddos potty trained at the same age/time. In my grandparent's era, children were toilet trained early (12-18 months). This had a lot to do with the needs of the adult, however, not necessarily the readiness of the child. Most American families are now waiting until their child is at least twenty-four months or beyond to introduce potty training. Keep in mind, that times are always changing!

An article by Healthy Children.org entitled "The Right Age to Potty Train", states that there is no exact right age potty train! Research over the past several decades indicates that there is no perfect age. Parents really need to look at the physical, mental, and emotional readiness of their child and go from there. These indicators could happen at vastly different ages.

Sumer Schmitt over at Giggles, Grace, and Naptime shares her experiences with potty training on "older toddler". Her son was nearly three and a half when he was fully potty trained. She shares her story of persevering through potty training and advises:

We, as moms, have heard it a million times. Don't compare. Don't compare your child to little Suzy down the street who was potty trained at 18 months. Or the story you read online about the 6 month old baby who is already doing elimination communication. Easier said than done, right? When you're in the thick of it though, it's hard not to get stuck in the comparison game.

Trust me, I get it. But, your child will potty train in his/her own time. Chances are, by the time your child reaches kindergarten, no one is even going to be talking about this milestone anymore. Just like they no longer talk about when your child first rolled over, sat up, crawled, or started walking. Those milestones are in the past and most children will all eventually catch up to one another.

Studies actually show that sometimes potty training later is better because your child will have a better developed vocabulary. Potty training may be easier and happen faster the later the age!

3.6 How to potty train your kid as a dad

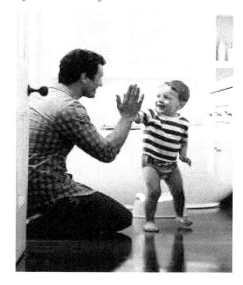

As a father, either single father or not our child is more likely to understand potty use if he's no longer wearing a nappy. Training pants are absorbent underwear worn during toilet training. They're less absorbent than nappies but are useful for holding in bigger messes like accidental poos. Once your child is wearing training pants, dress her in clothes that are easy to take off quickly.

Pull-ups are very popular and are marketed as helpful for toilet training. It isn't clear that they actually help. But you can try them to help your child get used to wearing underwear.

Generally, cloth training pants are less absorbent than

pull-ups and can feel a little less like a nappy. Pull-ups might be handier when you're going out. Wearing training pants is a big move for your child. If you celebrate it, the transition will be easier. Talk about how grown-up he is and how proud of him you are. I've heard all the tricks stickers, bribing with toys, special underpants. But you have to pick something that's consistent with your parenting style. I didn't use rewards elsewhere, so I didn't want to start here. What did work: Lots of undivided attention, positive reinforcement, love, affection and pride when my kids were successful. Making a big deal about small steps of progress is key. I didn't use any special stuff—no kiddie toilets, potty rings, or even pull-ups— because the local YMCA where my daughters attended didn't believe in them. We even had to sign a contract stating that we'd follow their potty training policy at home. I was instructed to just put the kids (they were around 2 1/2) on our regular toilet throughout the day when I thought they had to go. After a week and lots of "Yeah! You did number two!" and "Good for you! You made a wee-wee!" they were done, with barely any accidents. All told, I think they were just developmentally ready.

"The key is consistency," says James Singer, father of two, and a member of the Huggies Pull-Ups Potty Training Partners. "Whatever you do at home with your potty training plan, you also need to do elsewhere. For instance, if your child prefers to read a book while on the potty, talk to your daycare provider about sending in a favorite book. Keep in mind that daycare centers may be too busy to customize potty training to each child. In that case, ask them how they think they can help foster the success you have had at home and compromise. Then bring home something that works at daycare. If your child loves the soap they use at school, get some for home.

Boost the fun factor of using the potty with a Pee-Kaboo Reusable Potty Training Sticker. Slap a blank sticker onto the base of a portable potty, have your toddler pee in the potty, and then let him watch as an image of a train, flower, fire truck, or butterfly appears! After you empty, clean, and dry the potty, the image disappears, ready to be used again and again for up to six weeks. Too good to be true? We tested it on a formerly reluctant potty trainer, 2-year-old Gwenyth Mencel, who now shouts "Butterfly, butterfly!" when it's time to hit the potty. Are you counting down the days to the toilet transition? Or maybe you've already dabbled in a few less-than-successful attempts? Either way, we heard one thing again and again: Your kid has to be good and ready. And don't worry, he will be someday. "No child is going to graduate high school in diapers," says Carol Stevenson, a mom of three from Stevenson Ranch, California, who trained each one at a different age. "But it's so easy to get hung up and worried that your child's a certain age and not there yet, which adds so much pressure and turns it into a battle." Once you're convinced your kid's ready to ditch the diapers (watch for signs like showing an interest in the bathroom, telling you when she has to go, or wanting to be changed promptly after pooping), try any of these tricks to make it easier.

3.7 An explanation from an experience Dad

My wife, MJ, and I ran into the usual parent challenges when trying to potty-train our son. At first Will, then 2, was confused, then afraid, and next defiant. At 2 1/2 he still loved that diaper, and the mere sight of a toilet sent

him into a tantrum. The most frustrating part was that I knew he was ready. He would stay dry the entire night, wake up, and pee into his diaper while standing right in front of us, grinning. It was a not-so-subtle reminder that if Will was going to learn, it would be on his own terms.

MJ and I spent countless hours trying to make the bathroom more appealing. We brought Will's stuffed animals in there, let him flip through his books while sitting on the potty (good training for when he's older, like Dad), and even threw Cheerios in the bowl to give him a target. Nothing worked.

At last we got Will to stand on the stool, lift up the seat, pull his pants down, and loom over the toilet. But he still wouldn't go. "Dad, it's not working," he'd say in the cutest way imaginable.

At first I urged him to keep trying. No go. So I turned on the faucet, thinking the sound of running water would make him feel like peeing. But I forgot that he doesn't like noise, so this move merely upset him.

Finally I had a eureka moment. "Hey, Bud, how 'about if Dad pees with you, and we race?" I said. This clearly sparked Will's competitive spirit, because he brightened

up and agreed to the challenge. I shifted his stool to the right so I could squeeze in next to him, and we prepared for our duel. I told him we'd fire on the count of three. But my little cheater jumped the gun. I didn't even get to "two" before he let loose a stream into the toilet. Victory. Will giggled and grinned with pride, and I silently awarded myself first place in the "Best Dad in the Universe" contest for solving the potty-training riddle. I smiled broadly at father and son sharing a moment, hitting a milestone (er, Cheerio), and having some genuine fun.

A little too much fun, as it turns out. Will became so excited and began laughing so hard that he started falling in mid-spritz. I was still peeing as well, so I did my best to keep him balanced, all the while making sure we hit the porcelain bull's-eye.

Will's left foot slipped off the stool. I was able to catch him somewhat with my hip and right hand, but not before he instinctively turned toward me. Yup, that's right he sprayed me. A good father would've taken the punishment. But I'm squeamish, so I jerked my body away from his shower. That caused my own pee to hit the wall and ricochet onto my poor son's back.

We both fell to the floor, shocked and disgusted. We were silent for a moment, until Will spoke.

"Dada?" he said quizzically. "Yes, Bud?"

"You peed on me."

"To be fair, you peed on me first."

The two of us started cracking up belly laughs, guffaws, cackling, you name it - to such a degree that I would have peed myself right there if I hadn't just soaked my toddler. The racket attracted the attention of MJ, who came rushing over. When she turned the corner she stared at us: our soaked clothes, the yellow droplets slowly making their way down the wall.

I launched into an explanation. "Honey, you see, there was a pee race ..."

"I don't care," she interrupted, turning on her heels and walking away. "Just clean it up."

I did, and that day turned out to be a breakthrough. Will began using the toilet regularly (he asked me many times to race him again, but I never accepted) and was fully trained less than two months later. The bad news? He can't

resist the urge to tell anyone and everyone about the time Dad peed on him.

3.8 How to Potty train a kid as a grandpa

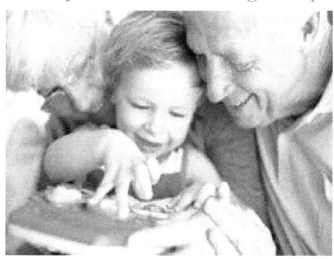

Potty training is one of the more difficult endeavors we face as old parents. Every child is different and has their own unique challenges.

Unfortunately, it's a messy, stinky destination that you'll quickly want to conquer, but will seemingly get stuck in the mud (no pun intended). So why do some grand parents struggle so much with potty training? The answer may be in the diversity, or lack there of our teachings. The way I see it, the more activities you do to promote potty usage, the better your child's chance of

success. You have to stack the deck in your favor. Some parents only do one or two things like buy pull-ups and

attempt to put their child on the potty until they get frustrated from it not working. There is a better way. In fact, several different ways which should all be used in conjunction to make potty time a little less night marish and actually more successful!

Children are typically ready to potty train around the ages of 2 or 3 but maybe earlier if there are older siblings to learn from. Look for the signs.

Look out for signs that your child is ready. These include pulling their diaper on and off, going a while or whole nap with a dry diaper, telling you they're going, showing curiosity about the potty and what goes in it, and going number 2 the same time each day.

When starting, dedicate 1-2 weeks to potty training. This includes pausing play-dates, car rides, outdoor activities, and basically anything that brings your child out of the house. Once you start, there's no turning back. Make sure you're in it for the long haul...all or nothing. Avoid pull-ups during the day as they give children a crutch to go, just like a diaper. Instead, let them be naked and

rush them to the potty if they start to go while saying, "Make sure you go pee pee in the potty."

Put them on the potty every 15 to 30 minutes. A lot of kids also have a set time of day when they do their "number 2" business. Make sure to put your child on the potty for several minutes during this time of day and encourage them to go number 2.

Make it enticing and convenient for them to go by providing a smaller, fun themed potty that's not so intimidating to a toddler. My son had a fire truck potty that he loved and we kept it in the room he would play in. Teach the process of going potty and washing hands with books! There are a ton of great books that you can read to your toddler while sitting on the potty.

Make a cool potty earning chart with fun stickers and rewards. My son received a sticker every time he went potty and after eight stickers he received a little cheap toy like a matchbox car. You can also reward with a few mini M&Ms when they're successful. Charts are a great way to be consistent. Nighttime potty training usually comes later. We put nighttime pull-ups on our toddler for a good six months after he was day time potty trained. It wasn't until he started going the entire night

without incident did we stop using them. Try your best to stay calm, use positive reinforcement, and not get angry or frustrated when they have an accident. You don't want your child to be anxious or stressed with potty time. Don't make them feel bad for having an accident. They might not tell you when it happens the next time.

As stated earlier, potty training is one of the most difficult parts of being a parent. Consistency is your friend in this situation. Don't give up. Even with hard work, regression is possible and normal. Keep working at it until your little one is a potty pro.

Chapter 4 How to potty train your kid in 3 days

The "Signs of Readiness"

I've heard people say that the child needs to show "signs of readiness" before you can potty train them for 3 days.

This is true. What most people don't understand is, "What exactly is a sign of readiness"? People often say that a sign of readiness is when the child starts showing interest in the toilet more than usual. In my opinion, this is an enormous misconception.

Children are curious creatures. As soon as they can crawl, they're out exploring their world. They inevitably find the toilet bowl and start playing in the water.

This is not "the sign" to look for (though it is if you want to prevent them from getting sick, hurt or causing other mayhem).

A necessary sign of potty training readiness is the ability for the child to frequently communicate his or her wants. I'm not talking about speech. I'm talking about gestures, behaviors, sounds, signing. If you can understand that a child wants something, and the child can direct you to the item, that is good enough.

Believe me, when a child is pulling your leg into the kitchen or bedroom, they know what they want, and they are effectively communicating with you! There is greater significance in this sign than you might think. What this behavior or attribute also means is that many children with Apraxia or speech, autism and other developmental problems can be potty trained using this method. Ultimately, the child learns that using the toilet is a good thing, something to be rewarded, and they will find a way to communicate their need to you. They like being rewarded.

A parent explained: My fifth child was diagnosed with Childhood Apraxia of Speech and was potty trained at 22 months old in under 3 days using 3

Day potty training method this is not an easy task. At the time his vocabulary consisted mainly of sounds - not actual words. If a child with apraxia can use potty at 22 month why did you think your own kid cant do that.

Secondly, your child must be able to go to bed without a bottle or cup, preferably two to three hours before bedtime.

4.1 There are a couple reasons why I say this.

1)I care about your child's dental health 2)It makes for easy potty training

What happens to you when you have a lot to drink just before going to bed? Late night visits to the bathroom! The same goes for your child. If you give them lots of fluid before bed, there's little chance they will wake up dry.

4.2 A few common questions I get from moms about this sign of readiness:

1)Our dinner is only an hour before bed, do I not give my child anything to drink? It is just fine for you to give your child something to drink with dinner. Just be sure that he's not getting tons just before he goes down for the night.

2)My child really enjoys his cup of milk before bed as it is part of our night time routine. Do I really need to stop this? No, you can continue as you have milk with your night time routine but try to decrease the amount. To do this maybe you can get him a smaller cup and then only

fill it half way full. Also be sure to follow the night time routine outlined in this eBook.

3)My child wakes often during the night needing a drink, I don't want to tell him no because it's really dry where we live. You can go ahead and let your child have his "sips" of water during the night if he really needs this but there is no need for full cups of water. Being that your child does wake for drinks, he shouldn't have a problem also getting up to go to the bathroom.

Third, in order for this method to work for children under the age of 22 months of age, your child must be waking up dry. Check for dryness within half an hour of them waking up. Don't wait until they've been up for an hour or so. By then, they will have peed and you won't get an accurate indication of readiness. If your child is over the age of 22 months old he should be waking up dry but don't worry too much if he does not. Just be sure to follow the night time method outlined in the eBook to help him with waking up dry.

4.3 A few common questions I get from moms about this sign of readiness:

1)My child is 3 years old and still wakes up with a full

diaper. Can I still potty training my child? Yes! As stated above, if your child or grandchild is over the age of 22 months and they still wake up wet, it's ok. Just be sure to follow the night time steps outlined in the eBook.

2)My first child is 5 years old and still wets the bed, I don't think my 2 year old will be able to be potty trained for nights. Can I just potty train for the days and use a pull-up or diaper for nights? Why would you want to? There is no need. You can easily potty train your child (even your older child) to wake up dry if you follow the method outlined in the eBook. It works!

3) My child is 18 months old and shows most the signs of readiness but doesn't wake up dry; can I still start potty training? Yes, just be sure to follow the steps outlined in the eBook for night time. I do recommend waiting until your child is 22 months of age because it can take longer than three days when they are younger than 22 months, but the choice is yours. It is my experience that children 22 months of age are at the ideal age to be

potty trained. It is entirely possible that a 15 month old shows these signs. For me, if my 15 month old showed these signs, I would still wait until 22 months.

4.4 The First day Journey to the 3 days potty training

Day 1 is the day that we decide to start potty training. First of all, as mentioned earlier, make sure that not only you, but also your child and anyone else who's involved, gets a good night's rest. This is extremely important. It's very difficult to accomplish something when you are not only tired but the child is tired and everyone is cranky.

It is on this day that you get rid of the diapers and the child starts wearing big boy and big girl underwear fulltime... There are no more diapers in this process... Now, some of you are saying, "Well, maybe we'll go ahead and use pull-ups or padded underwear." What I like to say is, "A diaper is a diaper no matter what you call it or what you disguise it as." And subconsciously, if you put the diaper on the child, it gives them the wrong message.

Also, seeing as that we've already explained how difficult this process is for the parents or the potty trainer as it is for the child, not having the diaper makes the parent or the potty trainer more vigilant. You will pay more attention if you know that the child does not have a diaper on.

For example, if you know the child has a diaper and you are out and about somewhere in a store or going out shopping you might say to yourself, "Well, we don't have to find a bathroom right now. We're kind of in a rush. You've got a diaper on." But note that the one time you tell that child that it's okay to go potty in that diaper; you have opened Pandora's Box. You've just told them, "its okay". And they will continue to do that and you will hit a lot of regressions. So, we start with allowing them to pick their big boy or girl underwear and put it on. (This is something you might have done during the pre-potty training process).

Then, you're going to sit down with your child and explain the process to them again. You can say, "Here's what we are doing; here is what Mommy expects; and here is what's going to happen." Then, you'll want to let them pick the spot for their potty chair.

You'll ask them, "Where do you want your potty chair?" We want to give them some control as well. If you have 2 bathrooms in the house, let them pick their favorite bathroom if they're going to be using the bathroom instead of the potty chair.

Then, you're going to take them to the bathroom. They are going to sit on the toilet and you are going to say, "Okay, Mommy wants you to use the bathroom." By this point, they should have seen you use the bathroom, so you can also say, "We want you to use the bathroom just like Mommy uses the bathroom." Don't be disappointed if nothing comes out. The act that getting them to sit there is a reward or it's an accomplishment all on its own. Once they get off the toilet, you're going to set a timer for 20 minutes.

Every 20 minutes for the first 3 days or for the first few days until they're trained, you are going to have them go and sit in the bathroom. When the timer goes off (and this is very important) it almost has to become a celebration in the house. Everybody can clap or say, "It's potty time. It's potty time. Let's go potty." And everyone can run to the bathroom.

Even with our older kids when we were potty training our youngest, would join into the celebration and run to the bathroom. And it was as if it was Cinco de Mayo or some big festivity in the house. That is very important because we're trying to make this a fun experience for the child.

Every time they go to the bathroom at those 20 minute intervals, you want to make sure they sit on the toilet for 3 to 5 minutes. This is not about them sitting on the toilet for hours; it's sitting on the toilet for 3 to 5 minutes. If they go right away and they pee or they do number 2, then they can get up right away.

Now, if they don't do either one then you want to make sure you wait the full 5 minutes with them sitting on the toilet. Note: At this point, we are not so much concerned about number 2. We want you and them to master number 1 first and then we'll move on. Now, even if they don't go, that is okay because the fact that you're getting them to sit down on the toilet is, again, an accomplishment all in its own.

But something that you want to see happen every single time they sit down on the toilet is for them to push. Even if they don't go number 2 or they don't do number 1, you want to make sure they push. So, you'll want to say, "Mommy wants to see you push. Now push." And some parents have told us, "Well, I can't tell when they're pushing." What you want to do is look at their stomach.

You can tell by the stomach muscle flexing whether they

are pushing or not. You see, with a child, it is impossible for them to hold and push at the same time. So, you're almost tricking them into using the potty by asking them to push. So, no matter what—no matter where you go, no matter what time it is—the minute they sit on the toilet you want to make sure that they push and they push every single time. Even if nothing comes out, as long as they push, that is a good thing because we want to get them used to using those muscles and pushing and moving whatever is inside of their system out. If you find they do not understand what pushing is, what you can do is just tickle their stomachs and the tickling sensation will cause them to contract their stomach muscles, which is a natural way to push.

The other thing that you want to start doing is giving them more fluids. Many people think that potty training is about not wetting themselves. That is not what potty training is about. Potty training is about recognizing when you have to go and knowing where to do it. So, one of the things that you're going to do to help them recognize that is giving them more fluids. However, you do not want to give them more juice because sometimes the sugar and starches that are in the juice can cause

constipation and other problems. Instead, you want to give them liquids like water and things that are going make them want to go potty. In addition to helping them potty, water also helps in the number 2 process as well, which we'll talk about later.

Now, sometimes what happens is that the child will sit for 5 minutes, they won't go, they'll get up and then they might wet themselves within a minute or two. So, here's what you do in that situation: shorten the amount of time that they sit on the toilet. Instead of sitting on the toilet for 5 minutes, let them sit on the toilet for 1 or 2 minutes, but you increase the frequency of how many times they go to the bathroom. So, instead of every 20 minutes, now it's every 15 minutes for 1 to 2 minutes. Another thing you'll want to do is ask them from the minute they get off the toilet and at least 3 or 4 times during that 20 minute timeframe, "Do you have to go potty? "Most of the time, they're going to tell you, "No," and that's okay.

You just want to get them used to hearing the words, "Do you have to go potty?" Then, when the 20 minutes are up and it's time to go potty, now the question is not, "Do you have to go potty?" Now, it's, "Time to potty."

One is asking and one is telling. Hopefully you see and understand the difference between the two statements. It's very, very important especially for psychologically getting the child to want to go and use the toilet.

4.5 Constipation

Alright, let's start with holding. Some children will actually hold number 2. Sometimes they will hold number 2 for a day or two days. When it finally becomes too painful they will let it all out into the diaper. First of all if you find your child is holding it that long and all the other methods are not working, and then put a diaper on to let them go. Holding bowel that long is not good for them. This is one of the rare times we recommend putting on a diaper. The thing to realize is...if they are holding it that long, then theoretically just by the nature of what potty training is, that says your child is potty trained and know what to do. For whatever reason they are afraid of the potty.

It's not an issue of potty training. It's an issue of being afraid or maybe going potty is too painful for them. If you find that their stool is hard, then it will lead to painful bowel movement. If they associate all bowels as

painful then they would rather hold the stool then to let it go. So the things that you can do are give them foods that will cause them to go to the bathroom. Give them more liquids (preferably water, not soda or juice), more liquids in their system the easier for them to go number You want to also do other things. When they're sitting on the toilet try to take their mind off the potty. Some ways to do that would be to rub their stomach or their feet. In the scientific world this is called neuro-linguistic programming. Basically you are trying to get their mind off of something that they're afraid of. So by doing something that feels good to them, you are associating the toilet with something that feels good. Now they're not afraid of that anymore. You want to tickle them. When you tickle them, it forces them to push. You've heard me use the word push over and over so it's something that I'm going to stress. Make sure they push. As long as they push you are doing good. They cannot hold and push at the same time. I cannot stress enough how important pushing is. If you feel they don't know what pushing is, then tickle their stomach and that will help them understand what pushing is. The other thing that you want to look at when it comes number 2 is constipation. There are a lot of things that cause constipation. Some causes of constipation are medical, while other causes are more mental. If you find your child is constipated, you want to do what I call the "bicycle trick". Don't ask how we had figured this out, but this works 100% of the times. What you do is you lay your child on their back. You should kneel in front of your child at the base of their feet.

Their feet should be almost touching your lap. Grab the base of their feet. Then rotate their legs as if they're riding a bicycle. Do this for about 10 minutes. Within 25 -30 minutes of doing this, the child will use the bathroom. We've told many parents to do this. Every parent I've told to try this, we've gotten a 100% success rate, whereas the child will end up using the bathroom within 30 minutes of doing the "bicycle trick".

So that is the constipation, and if you find the constipation lasting 4 or 5 days you may want to seek some form of medical attention for the child. That is not normal for them to be able to hold it for that many days.

4.6 The second day journey of the 3 days

Alright, so you've graduated from number 1. Your child

is doing very well using number 1. Now, it's time for them to start using number 2. There is not much difference between training them from number 1 to number 2. As a matter of fact, I would go so far to tell you that number 1 is a lot harder than number 2, and the reason being that when they go number 1, they have to actually take action to hold it inside.

In other words, for them not to wet themselves, they have to actually squeeze the sphincter muscle and hold the fluids inside. Whereas with number 2, they don't have to do anything to hold it. They actually have to push it out so it is an action that is a lot less difficult than holding the number 1 is. This is behaviour. They have to actually take a step. They have to be proactive to go number 2 so they have a whole lot more control in the number 2 process than they do in number 1. Now, again, one of the things that we want to make sure we do when they're sitting on the toilet is pushing. And, hopefully you understand how important the pushing strategy is. No matter how far along in the potty training process—whether they are two years old or whether they are four and a half—pushing is extremely important because that is how they are training themselves to go.

This is especially true when it comes to number 2. Now, some kids will want to go in number 2 in their diaper or a pull up. They will actually go and ask their parent for a pull up or a diaper to go number 2. Now, if this is the case for you, what you want to realize is the pull up then becomes a security blanket for the child.

In this case, what you might say is something to the effect of, "Okay, if you go number 2, then we'll put the pull up on." What that says is, "If you go number 2 first then we'll get

the pull up." Now, something else I've had parents do is actually go get the pull up, let them put the pull up on only around their ankles. That way, they have their security blanket on, and they can feel it, and they can see it, yet they're sitting on the toilet. This allows them to use the bathroom and feel comfortable.

The other thing you want is to make sure that you give them is more fluids as I explained earlier. And you will also want to make sure to track their schedule. A lot of kids will go to the bathroom for number 2 at the same time or around the same time every day. With my youngest son, it was like clockwork. Within 30 minutes of him eating anything, he would go to use the potty and

do number 2. So, we always knew after he ate that he was going to use the bathroom. Using a potty training journal is helpful.

If you don't have a potty journal and a potty chair or a potty chart, you can get yourself a potty training chart and journal to track when they go to the bathroom. Let's say you find that they go after dinner, which is around the time frame of 7:00 in the evening. Well, what happens is you're still using the same consistency as using number 1 which is every 20 minutes except now you are watching for 7 o'clock to come around because you know that they're going to be using the bathroom within a half hour.

At this point, what you want to do is time the bathroom use. You want to get them on the toilet but you also want to make sure that they stay on the toilet long enough to use the bathroom or use the bathroom to do number 2. their underwear again. It's going to help them make sure they use the bathroom the next time they go.

4.7 When they finally get it right

Alright, now you're taking them to the bathroom every

20 minutes and you go 3 days and you are not getting any accidents. Don't make the mistake that most parents make as I mentioned very early on. This is the stage when many parents decide that, "My child is potty trained and there was nothing left for me to do." This is the point in time where you want to be more consistent, more consistent, and more consistent.

This is when you want to make sure that you are still taking them to the bathroom every 20 minutes or you might change the interval from 20 minutes to 30 minutes. You might even feel comfortable waiting even longer than that - maybe 45 minutes. But don't let 45 minutes to an hour go by that you are not taking your child to the bathroom. Let me give you an example why this is. Your body has to get what's called "muscle memory." Remember at this point the child is only in stage 3 of potty training.

That's where they know what they're doing. They know what's wrong but they're thinking about it. It's not subconscious yet. At this point in time, the child is still thinking, "Should I go; should I not go? Where should I go? What should I do?" Think about it this way: Michael Jordan is one of the best basketball players that have

ever played the game, yet even when he was scoring 30, 40, 50 points a game, he was still shooting and practicing for hours a day, taking 500 to 600 foul shots every single day. Even though he was the best there was, he was still practicing harder than anybody else.

That is the difference between regular athletes and professionals. The professionals, they practice harder than anybody else because when they get into a situation, they do not have to think about it, the body automatically reacts. So, that's why when your child is finally starting to get it, you have to then make sure you maintain the consistency.

Chapter 5 Getting them to tell you

How do you get them to start telling you? Basically the question is how do we get your child from Stage 3 to Stage 4? And Stage 4 is where they can go to the bathroom themselves. They recognize on their own, they don't need you to take them to the bathroom every 20 minutes. Basically, its complete autonomy and freedom for the child and complete autonomy and freedom for you... So, the question is, "How do we get to that stage?" With consistency. You have to be consistent.

Once they start to show you they are ready, you have to make sure that you are continually being consistent. The other thing you can do is you can play the game that I call the "let's race to the potty game." All you do is sit at the table with your child and you say, "Okay, let's see who can get to the potty first and whoever wins gets a prize." So, basically it's a race between you and the child, and, of course, you're going to let the child win (but they don't know that).

Then, you pick a good reward of something that they're going to enjoy or really like. To start the race they have to say the words, "Mommy, I have to go potty." That's the cue. It's like saying "1, 2, 3, set go." But instead of

saying "1, 2, 3, set go," they say, "Mommy I have to go potty". Once they say that, the race begins, so the both of you run to the bathroom and the first one that gets to the bathroom wins the game. What this does is gets the child used to saying, "I have to go potty," and then the next steps are them going to the bathroom.

You want to practice this probably two or three times a day once you find that they are starting to be more consistent with no accidents. You don't want to start this game while they're in the potty training process because they've got enough to worry about. So, you want to start this only after you've seen that they have finally gotten it and they're starting to do pretty well on their own.

5.1 How to Use Positive Practice for Accidents

Another useful technique is positive practice for accidents. Dr. Schaefer describes this as what you should do when your child has an accident and wets or soils himself.

This technique involves firmly telling your child what he has done, taking him to the potty where he can clean and change himself (although you will likely need to

help) and then having him practice using the potty. Dr. Schaefer recommends going through the usual steps of using the potty at least five times, starting when "the child walks to the toilet, lowers his pants, briefly sits on the toilet (3 to 5 seconds), stands up, raises his pants, washes his hands, and then returns to the place where the accident occurred."

Although you are trying to teach him the consequences of having an accident, this should not take the form of punishment.

5.2 Children Tantrums

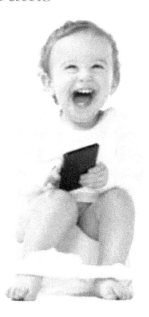

Tantrums are going to happen. A tantrum is frustration. That's the child not being able to verbally explain or talk about their emotion. So, the only way they know how to do that is through screaming and pitching a fit. Here's how you handle a tantrum... What you don't want to do is make potty training a battle. It's not a battle between you and the child, but the child is trying to battle you.

The child is trying to be in charge, and you're trying to be in charge at the same time. So, sometimes the way that you handle that is to totally ignore the tantrum. If your child is throwing a tantrum, you can walk away and say, "Mommy is not listening to you. Mommy will talk to you when you are calmed down," or "Mommy is not listening to you when your voice is louder than Mommy's." So you can turn around and use reverse psychology by turning the tables on your child. Once they have calmed down, you will want to say in a very strong and direct voice, "Mommy did not appreciate that," or "Grandma did not appreciate that," or "Daddy did not appreciate that behavior.

We expect better things. Let's go and try again." So, now you go right back to the basics and you take the child back to the bathroom and say, "We are going to use the bathroom and here's what we expect." If they throw a tantrum again, you walk away.Mind you, while

that tantrum is going on, do not give them any rewards. Do not allow them to play with their toys. They are not allowed to do any of that fun stuff that they normally would want to do because you want to associate that tantrum with a bad behavior that results in loosing something.

So, the most important thing I can tell you is to ignore the tantrum, don't pay attention to it because as the laws of physics say, "For every action, there's an equal and opposite reaction." If you react to that tantrum, they are going to react to you. Once you react, they react. You react again, they react and it's going to escalate even more.

So, the easiest way to squash it is not to put in the energy toward that tantrum. Once the child feels and sees that they're not getting energy out of you, then they realize that they're getting nothing by throwing this tantrum and there's nothing to be gained from it.

5.3 Regression in potty Training

What is a regression? A regression is a child that was potty trained, they were doing well, or they were starting to do well and for whatever reasons, they have

done an about-face. Now, they are wetting themselves or they are soiling their diapers with poop. The question is "What really is the regression? What are the cause and the root of that regression?" These are the issues that need to be dealt with. Usually a regression is not so much an issue with potty training, but it's an emotional issue. The child will regress as a way to get attention or as a way of expression.

So, most parents deal with regression by dealing with potty training, but the reality is the best way to deal with a regression is to try to find the underlying root cause. It could be one of many things causing the regression. A new baby being born, you've moved, a friend has moved, a family member might have passed away... Something has happened in that child's life and they don't know how to express it except through regression.

Something that a lot of parents have asked is, "When it comes to potty training, we've got a new baby on the way, should I wait to have the baby or will they regress if I potty train them and then we have the baby?" The best thing to do is to potty train them now. It is a lot easier to retrain a child that has been trained and has

gone through a regression than it is to try to train a child that has never been trained. In addition to that as a parent, if you are having a new baby coming, you do not want to have a new baby and potty training duties at the same time. That's very, very, difficult. What I always tell parents is that they'll only need two to three days to get the child to Stage 3. Stage 4 is what will take you a couple of days from there. Some kids even get to Stage 4 in one day.

But the key is, take the two or three days, get your child to Stage 3, then through consistency, work toward getting them to Stage 4. When the new baby comes, or whatever that activity is—whether it's a vacation or a move—if they do regress, they've already been trained. Getting them back and reversing the regression is going to be a lot easier than if you had never started at all. So what you want to do when your child does regress is you go back to the basics. This includes them being on the toilet every 20 minutes for 3-5 minutes. They will continue to do that until they stop the regressive behavior.

The only time our youngest had a regression, I went on a business trip with Greg. Lorenzo had been fully potty

trained for about three months both day and night. Then I went on that business trip with my husband, and Lorenzo went to stay at Grandma's. We only were gone Thursday, Friday, and Saturday and came back on Sunday. When we returned, it was as if this child had never seen a potty chair or had been potty trained in his life. Now I have no idea what happened in those four days. Maybe Grandma had let him do whatever he wanted, I do not know. Or maybe he just said, "You know what? You guys left me, and I'm going to fix you guys." Basically, we took him back to the basics, went back to every 20 minutes with him on the toilet. And within about a day, he was back to normal. But it was a little scary seeing that happen.

5.4 Addressing fear in the kids

What you want to do is separate the difference between a fear of the toilet and potty training. Many of the parents that we have worked with have lumped the two into one category by saying that the fear of the toilet is a potty training problem. The reality is that a fear of the toilet has nothing to do with potty training, and, in most cases, it is a fear of the toilet as we noted earlier. So

what you have to do is address that fear by sitting and asking your child. Don't be afraid to do this. Just ask them what they are afraid of. Sometimes it might not be the potty training, but something else. One of the things that you can do to help your child if there is a fear of the toilet is get yourself a potty chair or potty seat insert. An insert is actually put into the toilet and the child can sit on that toilet instead of the adult seat, which is especially helpful if the child is a little bit smaller.

They are usually colorful and have giraffes on them and dinosaurs. There is also a handle so the child can hold on to the handle and balance themselves. This will help them feel safe and comfortable without the fear of falling into the toilet. Placing a step stool under their feet will also assist them in this area. But, if you find that they have a fear of the toilet, then a potty training chair will be the way to go instead of the insert.

Now the question is this, if there's a fear of the toilet, what is the cause of that fear? Sometimes it can be pain that the child has when they are going to the bathroom. This is especially true with number 2. So the question is, have they ever had diarrhea or have they ever had a diaper that was on too long which caused a skin

irritation? They are now associating the toilet and potty with that pain.

It might possibly be constipation. As an adult, constipation can be very painful. So, think about the child. It also might not be actual constipation, but some kids naturally have hard stools and letting that go can be extremely painful for them. If that is the case, you want to make sure that you take a look when your child does use the bathroom more if they are in their diaper. Is their stool harder or is it soft? Was there any illness like the stomach virus or anything that caused them some pain? These are all the things that can cause the child to be not only fearful of the toilet, but can also cause a child to regress. So you want to be careful about this and ask yourself whether any of this has happened.

If you find the child has hard stool, one of the things that you can do is start giving the child more water, less sugar, and less starchy items, which will help them become hydrated. When the body becomes dehydrated, it will start to pull any fluids that it can get wherever it can get it. One of the places that it pulls the fluid from is going to be the stomach and the intestines. And once those fluids are pulled out, the result is hardened stool.

Once that stool becomes hard it's going to be very difficult and very painful for that child to go to the bathroom. So having fluids in the system will help give him or her softer stool. Something else that you can do if there is a fear of the toilet is calling it by a different name. Instead of calling it "potty," you can give it another name that doesn't bear a negative connotation. Something simple might be, "Let's go push."

Another thing that will help you make the experience more enjoyable for the child is to place books by the toilet. You should also have some toys in the bathroom or let them

bring some toys with them so that it's a comfortable environment and something that is more fun for them. Again, the key is making it a loving time and not a stressful time. If you can read to them or let them look at picture books, it turns into more of an enjoyable process and a less stressful process.

5.5 Potty training Twins or multiple children

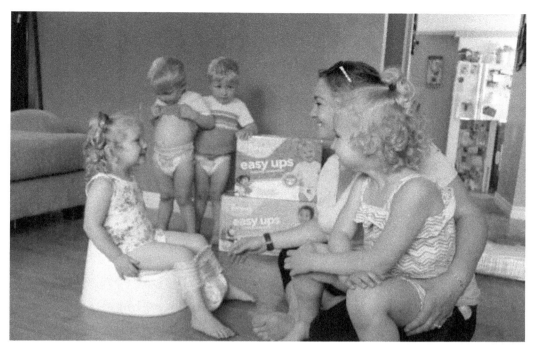

I have many parents with twins or multiples ask if this method can work for them. I also have parents with children at two different ages ask if the children can be potty trained simultaneously. The answer to both of these situations is "YES". You can potty train twins, multiples and two or more children at the same time. It's more demanding on you, and may take a few extra days, but it can be done.

If I, personally, had to choose between potty training multiples simultaneously or doing it one-at-a-time, I

would bite the bullet and do them all at the same time; "just be done with it." Having someone to help out is by far the best way. Be sure they read the guide. Discuss with them how you want situations handled. The two of you need to handle things identically. You can go it alone if you need to. Just be mentally prepared for some extra work. Also, the children must be right by your side at all times. If one child needs to use the restroom, ask the other child to come with. The underlying principle for potty training two or more children simultaneously is that you need to treat each child as an individual. Ideally, each child should have their own potty chair. They should each have their own underclothes and their own favorite treats and favorite drinks. Be sure to not use one's successes against the other child or children. Don't say things like, "See, Johnny can do it. Now you need to too." Just because one child might catch on right away doesn't mean that the other child / children will get it the first day or two. Keep in mind that they are individuals and that they may catch on at different times.

5.6 Help from daycare provider

If your child is in daycare be sure to discuss with your

daycare providers your plan a day or two before you start. Explain to them that when your child returns to daycare that they are not to put a pull-up or diaper on the child. They may come back to you and say that if the child has an accident, they will put a diaper on the child.

Gently remind them about the importance of being consistent, about how that would send mixed signals to the child, and could undo all the progress you've worked so hard to achieve, and that you greatly appreciate their support. Maybe even offer a pair of movie tickets. You or your spouse may need to take Friday or Monday off from work to give this method the best possible chance for success. Do not put your child in daycare during the three days. It's just too soon.

Day 4 is the earliest that I recommend returning your child to daycare.

Sometimes you may just have to play it by ear. At the end of day 3, if the whole toilet thing has not "clicked" with your child, you may need to take the next day off from work. The "clicking" or "getting it" needs to occur before the child returns to daycare. If your daycare provider is not on board with you then you might have a set back or two. I've never had my kids in daycare but

many of the moms that I've helped potty train have kids in daycare.

There are many wonderful daycare providers out there and they are willing to work with the parents but there are some that want nothing to do with helping the parents out. They want the child in a pull-up or diaper until they leave for school. If your daycare provider is one that isn't willing to support you during this training you might need to spend an extra day or two at home to make sure that there are no more accidents and that the child is confident in his new skill. You may need to be firm with your daycare provider with regards to your "no diaper" position.

If you are concerned about your daycare provider putting a pull-up or diaper back on your child, you might want to try Pods. Pods are little thin strips you place in your little ones underwear. These strips will absorb any accident your child has so he doesn't make a "mess" on the floor. Your child will feel the strips turn to a cold jell like substance and asked to go to the bathroom. The daycare provider can then just replace the strip. Pods can be the solution for those hard to work with daycare providers.

5.7 Travelling and Errands during potty Training

Alright, let's face the fact. You are a busy Mom or busy Dad or a busy Grandparent or a busy potty trainer. But you don't want to be stuck in the house during that potty training process. And yes —for a day or two you might be. But don't let potty training keep you from enjoying life and having fun and doing the things that you got to do.You may have shopping to do and errands to run. You might have a family to take care of. You've got things that you need to do. So here are some tips that will help you have a more successful potty training experience especially when you have things that you need to do.

First of all, you want to get yourself a spill-proof travel potty. If you don't have one, try to get one online travel and get yourself a spill-proof travel potty. Basically, it is a simple little potty chair which has a spill-proof lid. With that, you can keep it in the car so instead of having to be home to go to the bathroom every 20 minutes. You can be in the mall, you can be at the grocery store, you can be out shopping, and your child can still use the potty without the fear of having accidents. When you are

travelling or you're going to run errands, what you want to do is just like with the day care scenario, you want to use the bathroom before you leave. You will also want to plan your day and where you will be going so you'll be prepared about whether or not those places have bathrooms.

In other words, if you are going to place A and they have a bathroom and place B, does not have a bathroom, then you want to go to place B first right when you leave the house because your child has just gone. Once we would get to a location like a grocery store or a mall, especially if this is a grocery store or a mall that you've never been to, we would find the bathroom. So now, let's say we are out in the middle of shopping and Lorenzo had to go to the bathroom. It's wasn't a problem.

As soon as he said he had to go to the bathroom or we said, "Lorenzo, do you have to go to the bathroom?" and he said, "Yes," we knew where the bathrooms were. Most parents don't take that one step so what happens is the child says, "I have to go to the bathroom," the parents are in a state of panic to find the bathrooms. So, when we first got to the store, we would find the

bathroom and then go to the bathroom. We would then get our most important stuff done first because we knew we just went to the bathroom and had more free time now than we might later. So, the smaller, less important things could wait. Back to the travel potty, these are really great because they will also help you out when you are going to take a long road trip. If you don't have one, you know that stopping frequently is going to be an issue.

When Lorenzo was 2 years and 2 weeks, we had him fully potty trained and we took a trip to Florida. Back then, we were at Code Orange, and the government said it wasn't a good idea to fly. So, we decided to take a bus with three kids from Connecticut to Florida. It was a thirty-hour bus ride with a child that just finished potty training. To tell you it was a challenge is an understatement. Back then, there weren't spill-proof potty chairs so we didn't have one to bring, so we bought a huge 2 litre bottle. Every 20 minutes on the bus, we would hide in the corner or go into to the back and say, "Okay Lorenzo, pee into the bottle," and that's what he did. When he had to go number 2 luckily for us, was during a rest stop. But we didn't let the fact that he

had the potty train keep us from doing what we had to do.

Chapter 6 Naptime and Nighttime Training

6.1 Naptime

Yes it's ok to put your child down for a nap during training. I personally have found that most kids will not have an accident if you have them go pee before the nap and then just as they wake up. Make sure you stay close though so you know when your child wakes.

6.2 Nighttime

Do not give your child anything to drink when they are getting ready for bed. In fact, it's best to stop the liquids 2 to 3 hours beforehand. Take them to the toilet at least twice before tucking them in to bed for the night. If nothing happens in the bathroom, maybe read a book together for a few minutes and try again. Remember what I said about "trying" don't keep them on the toilet. Having them clear their bladder is important. Once your child has released twice you can put them in bed. Do not use a diaper (you shouldn't have any).

If your child has a hard time waking up dry and they are older than 22 months, the following procedure may help:

• Wake the child 1 hour after he or she has gone to sleep

• Take them to the toilet and return them to bed

• In the morning, wake the child 1 hour before they normally arise

Take them to the toilet This helps the child realize two things:

1) It is ok to get up to go pee

2) It is also expected If your child is in a crib, you can still follow these steps.

You just need to keep an ear open for them. If you hear your child stirring, or whimpering, they may need to pee. You do not need to do the above steps if your child usually wakes up dry. Your child may wet the bed at night. Don't be alarmed or upset.

This is halfway to be expected – we're giving them lots of liquid. Don't make a big deal of it – don't reprimand or scold. Just change the sheets. Remind the child to tell you when he needs to go pee, and that they need to keep their underwear dry. Again, don't be negative; don't say "Bad, No," etc.

This will be the end of a busy and perhaps frustrating day. Do not worry. It will click; your child will "get it", if

not tomorrow, then on the third day. Be sure to keep a positive and loving attitude with your child, even if you have to change sheets in the middle of the night.

A tip for parents with older children: To help your child to go to the bathroom before bed and to stay dry during the night you can try using a chart system with the following on it:

6.3 Bedtime Routine:

- go pee

- put on night clothes

- read a book

- brush teeth

- go pee again

- keep bed dry all night

Let your child know that if he gets a star by each one he will get a prize in the morning.

Remind him that he's got to get up and go pee if he's got to go. A special tip, that works for even the hardest of cases. The following has been used even with long time bed-wetters to help them overcome bed wetting... Once your child goes to sleep, make a bed up on the

floor without him knowing. Now throughout the night you will say to him "be sure to tell mommy when you

have to go pee". Anytime during the night when you hear him start to move and stir around, say to him "Do you have to go pee? Make sure tell mommy when you have to go pee".

What this does is allows you to see how often your child is stirring in his bed and will help him remember that he's suppose to pee in the potty not in his bed.

6.4 Toddler discipline and proper upbringing

Have you ever found yourself in deep negotiations with your 2-year-old over whether she can wear her princess costume to preschool for the fifth day in a row? Have you taken the "walk of shame" out of the local supermarket after your toddler threw a temper tantrum on the floor? There may be comfort in knowing you're not alone, but that doesn't make navigating the early years of discipline any easier.

Toddlerhood is a particularly vexing time for parents because this is the age at which children start to become

more independent and discover themselves as individuals. Yet they still have a limited ability to communicate and reason.

Child development specialist Claire Lerner, director of parenting resources for the nonprofit organization Zero to Three, says, "They understand that their actions matter -- they can make things happen. This leads them to want to make their imprint on the world and assert themselves in a way they didn't when they were a baby. The problem is they have very little self-control and they're not rational thinkers. It's a very challenging combination."

What do you do when your adorable toddler engages in not-so-adorable behavior, like hitting the friend who snatches her toy, biting Mommy, or throwing her unwanted plate of peas across the room? Is it time for...timeout?

Timeout -- removing a child from the environment where misbehavior has occurred to a "neutral," unstimulating space -- can be effective for toddlers if it's used in the right way, says Jennifer Shu, MD, an Atlanta pediatrician, editor of Baby and Child Health and co-author of Food Fights: Winning the Nutritional

 Challenges of Parenthood Armed With Insight, Humor, and a Bottle of Ketchup and Heading Home With Your Newborn: From Birth to Reality.

"Especially at this age, timeout shouldn't be punitive. It's a break in the action, a chance to nip what they're doing in the bud."

Timeouts shouldn't be imposed in anger, agrees Elizabeth Pantley, president of Better Beginnings, a family resource and education company in Seattle, and author of several parenting books, including The No-Cry Discipline Solution. "The purpose of timeout is not to punish your child but to give him a moment to get control and reenter the situation feeling better able to cope." It also gives you the chance to take a breath and step away from the conflict for a moment so you don't lose your temper.

6.5 Timeouts is Not for Every Kid

Some experts insist that timeouts work for all, but Shu and Pantley disagree. "For some kids who just hate to be alone, it's a much bigger punishment than it's worth, especially with young toddlers," says Shu. "They get so upset because you're abandoning them that they don't remember why they're there, and it makes things worse." She suggests holding a child with these fears in a bear hug and helping her calm down.

You can also try warding off the kind of behavior that might warrant a timeout with "time-in." That means noticing when your children's behavior is starting to get out of hand and spending five or 10 minutes with them before they seriously misbehave. "It's like a preemptive strike," Shu says. "Once they've gotten some quality time with you, you can usually count on reasonably OK behavior for a little while."

6.6 Toddler Discipline Dos & Don'ts

Shu says a good stage to initiate timeouts is when your toddler is around age 2. Here are a few guidelines.

Do remove your child from the situation. Do tell him what the problem behavior was.

Use simple words like "No hitting. Hitting hurts."

Don'tberateyourchild.

Do place her in a quiet spot -- the same place every time, if possible. For young toddlers, this may have to be a play yard or other enclosed space.

Don't keep him there long—the usual rule of thumb is one minute per year of age. Do sit down with your child after timeout is over and reassure her with a hug while you "debrief" by saying something like, "We're not going to hit anymore, right?" Don't belabor what the child did wrong. Instead, ask her to show you how she can play nicely.

6.7 Commandments Discipline for Toddler

Children aren't born with social skills it's human nature for them to start out with a survival-of-the-fittest mentality. That's why you need to teach your toddler how to act appropriately and safely -- when you're around and when you're not. In a nutshell, your job is to implant a "good citizen" memory chip in her brain (Freud called this the superego) that will remind her how she's supposed to behave. It's a bit like breaking a wild horse, but you won't break your child's spirit if you do it correctly. The seeds of discipline that you plant now will blossom later, and you'll be very thankful for the fruits of your labor. (Just don't expect a tree to grow overnight.) Here are the commandments you should

commit to memory.

1. Expect rough spots. Certain situations and times of the day tend to trigger bad behavior. Prime suspect

   number 1: transitions from one activity to the next (waking up, going to bed, stopping play to eat dinner). Give your child a heads-up so he's more prepared to switch gears ("After you build one more block tower, we will be having dinner").

2. Pick your battles. If you say no 20 times a day, it will lose its effectiveness. Prioritize behaviors into large, medium, and those too insignificant to bother with. In Starbucks terms, there are Venti, Grande, and Tall toddler screwups. If you ignore a minor infraction -- your toddler screams whenever you check your e-mail -- she'll eventually stop doing it because she'll see that it doesn't get a rise out of you.

3. Use a prevent defense. Sorry for the football cliche, but this one is easy. Make your house kid-friendly, and have reasonable expectations. If you clear your Swarovski crystal collection off the end table, your child won't be tempted to fling it at the TV set. If you're taking your family out to dinner, go early so you won't have to wait for a table.

4. Make your statements short and sweet. Speak in brief sentences, such as "No hitting." This is much more effective than "Chaz, you know it's not nice to hit the dog." You'll lose Chaz right after "you know."

5. Distract and redirect. Obviously, you do this all day. But when you try to get your child interested in a different activity, she'll invariably go back to what she was doing -- just to see whether she can get away with it. Don't give up. Even if your child unrolls the entire toilet-paper roll for the 10th time today, calmly remove her from the bathroom and close the door.

6. Introduce consequences. Your child should learn the natural outcomes of his behavior -- otherwise known as cause and effect. For example, if he loudly insists on selecting his pajamas (which takes an eternity), then he's also choosing not to read books before bed. Cause: Prolonged picking = Effect: No time to read. Next time, he may choose his pj's more quickly or let you pick them out.

7. Don't back down to avoid conflict. We all hate to be the party pooper, but you shouldn't give in just to escape a showdown at the grocery store. If you decide

that your child can't have the cereal that she saw on TV, stick to your guns. Later, you'll be happy you did.

8. Anticipate bids for attention. Yes, your little angel will act up when your attention is diverted (making dinner,

talking on the phone). That's why it's essential to provide some entertainment (a favorite toy, a quick snack). True story: My son once ate dog food while I was on the phone with a patient. Take-home lesson: If you don't provide something for your toddler to do when you're busy, she'll find something -- and the results may not be pretty.

9. Focus on the behavior, not the child. Always say that a particular behavior is bad. Never tell your child that he is bad. You want him to know that you love him, but you don't love the way he's acting right now.

10. Give your child choices. This will make her feel as if she's got a vote. Just make sure you don't offer too many options and that they're all things that

you want to accomplish, such as, "It's your choice: You can put your shoes on first, or your coat."

11. Don't yell. But change your voice. It's not the volume, but your tone that gets your point across.

Remember The Godfather? Don Corleone never needed to yell.

12. Catch your child being good. If you praise your child when he behaves well, he'll do it more often -- and he'll be less likely to behave badly just to get your attention.

Positive reinforcement is fertilizer for that superego.

13. Act immediately. Don't wait to discipline your toddler. She won't remember why she's in trouble more than five minutes after she did the dirty deed.

14. Be a good role model. If you're calm under pressure, your child will take the cue. And if you have a temper tantrum when you're upset, expect that he'll do the same. He's watching you, always watching.

15. Don't treat your child as if she's an adult. She really doesn't want to hear a lecture from you and won't be able to understand it. The next time she throws her spaghetti, don't break into the "You Can't Throw Your Food" lecture. Calmly evict her from the kitchen for the night.

16. Use time-outs -- even at this age. Call it the naughty chair or whatever you like, but take your child away from playing and don't pay attention to him for one

minute for each year of age. Depriving him of your attention is the most effective way to get your message across. Realistically, kids under 2 won't sit in a corner or on a chair -- and it's fine for them to be on the floor kicking and screaming. (Just make sure the time-out location is a safe one.) Reserve time-outs for particularly inappropriate behaviors -- if your child bites his friend's arm, for example -- and use a time-out every time the offense occurs.

17. Don't negotiate with your child or make promises. This isn't Capitol Hill. Try to avoid saying anything like, "If you behave, I'll buy you that doll you want." Otherwise, you'll create a 3-year-old whose good behavior will always come with a price tag. (Think Veruca Salt from Charlie and the Chocolate Factory.)

18. Shift your strategies over time. What worked beautifully when your child was 15 months probably isn't going to work when he's 2. He'll have read your playbooks and watched the films.

19. Don't spank. Although you may be tempted at times, remember that you are the grown-up. Don't resort to acting like a child. There are many more effective ways of getting your message across. Spanking your child for

hitting or kicking you, for example, just shows him that it's okay to use force. Finally, if your toddler is pushing your buttons for the umpteenth time and you think you're about to lose it, try to take a step back. You'll get a better idea of which manipulative behaviors your child is using and you'll get a fresh perspective on how to change your approach.

20. Remind your child that you love her. It's always good to end a discipline discussion with a positive comment. This shows your child that you're ready to move on and not dwell on the problem. It also reinforces the reason you're setting limits -- because you love her.

6.8 Disciplining Your Toddler to make the right choice

As a 2-year-old, Nathaniel Lampros of Sandy, Utah, was fascinated with toy swords and loved to duel with Kenayde, his 4-year-old sister. But inevitably, he'd whack her in the head, she'd dissolve in tears, and Angela, their mother, would come running to see what had happened. She'd ask

Nathaniel to apologize, as well as give Kenayde a hug and make her laugh to pacify hurt feelings. If he resisted, Angela would put her son in

time-out.

"I worried that Nathaniel would never outgrow his rough behavior, and there were days when I'd get so frustrated with him that I'd end up crying," recalls Lampros, now a mother of four. "But I really wanted Nathaniel to play nicely, so I did my best to teach him how to do it."

For many mothers, doling out effective discipline is one of the toughest and most frustrating tasks of parenting, a seemingly never-ending test of wills between you and your child. Because just when your 2-year-old "gets" that she can't thump her baby brother in the head with a doll, she'll latch on to another bothersome behavior — and the process starts anew.

How exactly does one "discipline" a toddler? Some people equate it with spanking and punishment, but that's not what we're talking about. As many parenting experts see it, discipline is about setting rules to stop your little one from engaging in behavior that's aggressive (hitting and biting), dangerous (running out in the street), and inappropriate (throwing food). It's also about following through with consequences when he breaks the rules — or what Linda Pearson, a Denver-based psychiatric nurse practitioner who specializes in

family and parent counseling, calls "being a good boss." Here are seven strategies that can help you set limits and stop bad behavior.

1. Pick Your Battles

"If you're always saying, 'No, no, no,' your child will tune out the no and won't understand your priorities," says

Pearson, author of The Discipline Miracle. "Plus you can't possibly follow through on all of the nos.'" Define what's important to you, set limits accordingly, and follow through with appropriate consequences. Then ease up on little things that are annoying but otherwise fall into the "who cares?"

category—the habits your child is likely to outgrow, such as insisting on wearing purple (and only purple).

"Keeping a good relationship with your child—who is of course in reality totally dependent upon you—is more important for her growth than trying to force her to respond in ways that she simply is not going to respond," says Elizabeth Berger, M.D., child psychiatrist and author of Raising Kids with Character. You may worry that "giving in" will create a spoiled monster, but Dr. Berger says this common anxiety isn't justified.

For Anna Lucca of Washington, D.C., that means letting her 2-1/2-year-old daughter trash her bedroom before she dozes off for a nap. "I find books and clothes scattered all over the floor when Isabel wakes up, so she must get out of bed to play after I put her down," Lucca says. "I tell her not to make a mess, but she doesn't listen. Rather than try to catch her in the act and say,

'No, no, no,' I make her clean up right after her nap." Lucca is also quick to praise Isabel for saying please and sharing toys with her 5-month-old sister. "Hopefully, the positive reinforcement will encourage Isabel to do more of the good behavior—and less of the bad," she says.

2. Know Your Child's Triggers

Some misbehavior is preventable—as long as you can anticipate what will spark it and you create a game plan in advance, such as removing tangible temptations. This strategy worked for Jean Nelson of Pasadena, California, after her 2-year-old son took delight in dragging toilet paper down the hall, giggling as the roll unfurled behind him. "The first two times Luke did it, I told him, 'No,' but when he did it a third time, I moved the toilet paper to a high shelf in the bathroom that he couldn't reach," Nelson says. "For a toddler, pulling toilet paper is

irresistible fun. It was easier to take it out of his way than to fight about it."

If your 18-month-old is prone to grabbing cans off grocery store shelves, bring toys for him to play with in the cart while you're shopping. If your 2-year-old won't share her stuffed animals during playdates at home, remove them from the designated play area before her pal arrives. And if your 3-year-old likes to draw on the walls, stash the crayons in an out-of-reach drawer and don't let him color without supervision.

3. Practice Prevention

Some children act out when they're hungry, overtired, or frustrated from being cooped up inside, says Harvey Karp, M.D., creator of the DVD and book The Happiest Toddler on the Block. If your child tends to be happy and energetic in the morning but is tired and grumpy after lunch, schedule trips to the store and visits to the doctor for when she's at her best. Prepare her for any new experiences, and explain how you expect her to act.

Also prepare her for shifting activities: "In a few minutes we'll need to pick up the toys and get ready to go home." The better prepared a child feels, the less likely she is to make a fuss.

4. Be Consistent

"Between the ages of 2 and 3, children are working hard to understand how their behavior impacts the people around them," says Claire Lerner, LCSW, director of parenting resources with Zero to Three, a nationwide nonprofit promoting the healthy development of babies and toddlers. "If your reaction to a situation keeps changing—one day you let your son throw a ball in the house and the next you don't—you'll confuse him with mixed signals."

There's no timetable as to how many incidents and reprimands it will take before your child stops a certain misbehavior. But if you always respond the same way, he'll probably learn his lesson after four or five times. Consistency was key for Orly Isaacson of Bethesda, Maryland, when her 18-month-old went through a biting phase. Each time Sasha chomped on

Isaacson's finger, she used a louder-than-usual voice to correct her — "No, Sasha! Don't bite! That hurts Mommy!" — and then handed her a toy as a distraction. "I'm very low-key, so raising my voice startled Sasha and got the message across fast," she says. A caveat: by age 2, many kids learn how to make their parents lose resolve just by

being cute. Don't let your child's tactics sway you — no matter how cute (or clever) they are.

5. Don't Get Emotional

Sure, it's hard to stay calm when your 18-month-old yanks the dog's tail or your 3-year-old refuses to brush his teeth for the gazillionth night in a row. But if you scream in anger, the message you're trying to send will

get lost and the situation will escalate, fast.

"When a child is flooded with a parent's negative mood, he'll see the emotion and won't hear what you're saying," advised the late William Coleman, M.D., professor of pediatrics at the University of North Carolina Medical School in Chapel Hill. Indeed, an angry reaction will only enhance the entertainment value for your child, so resist the urge to raise your voice. Take a deep breath, count to three, and get down to your child's eye level. Be fast and firm, serious and stern when you deliver the reprimand.

Trade in the goal of "controlling your child" for the goal of "controlling the situation," advises Dr. Berger. "This may mean re-adjusting your ideas of what is possible for a time until your daughter's self-discipline has a chance to grow a little more," she says. "You may need to lower

your expectations of her patience and her self-control somewhat. If your goal is to keep the day going along smoothly, so that there are fewer opportunities for you both to feel frustrated, that would be a constructive direction."

6. Listen and Repeat

Kids feel better when they know they have been heard, so whenever possible, repeat your child's concerns. If she's whining in the grocery store because you won't let her open the cookies, say something like: "It sounds like you're mad at me because I won't let you open the cookies until we get home. I'm sorry you feel that way, but the store won't let us open things until they're paid for. That's its policy." This won't satisfy her urge, but it will reduce her anger and defuse the conflict.

7. Keep It Short and Simple

If you're like most first-time parents, you tend to reason with your child when she breaks rules, offering detailed explanations about what she did wrong and issuing detailed threats about the privileges she'll lose if she doesn't stop misbehaving. But as a discipline strategy, overt-talking is as ineffective as becoming overly

emotional, according to Dr. Coleman. While an 18-month-old lacks the cognitive ability to understand complex sentences, a 2- or 3-year-old with more developed language skills still lacks the attention span to absorb what you're saying.

Instead, speak in short phrases, repeating them a few times and incorporating vocal inflections and facial expressions. For example, if your 18-month-old swats

your arm, say, "No, Jake! Don't hit Mommy! That hurts! No hitting." A 2-year-old can comprehend a bit more: "Evan, no jumping on the sofa! No jumping. Jumping is dangerous—you could fall. No jumping!" And a 3-year-old can process cause and effect, so state the consequences of the behavior: "Ashley, your teeth need to be brushed. You can brush them, or I can brush them for you. You decide. The longer it takes, the less time we'll have to read Dr. Seuss."

8. Offer Choices

When a child refuses to do (or stop doing) something, the real issue is usually control: You've got it; she wants it. So, whenever possible, give your preschooler some control by offering a limited set of choices. Rather than

commanding her to clean up her room, ask her, "Which would you like to pick up first, your books or your blocks?" Be sure the choices are limited, specific, and acceptable to you, however. "Where do you want to start?" may be overwhelming to your child, and a choice that's not acceptable to you will only amplify the conflict.

9. Watch Your Words

It helps to turn "you" statements into "I" messages. Instead of saying, "You're so selfish that you won't even

share your toys with your best friend," try "I like it better when I see kids sharing their toys." Another good technique is to focus on do's rather than don'ts. If you tell a 3-year-old that he can't leave his trike in the hallway, he may want to argue. A better approach: "If you move your trike out to the porch, it won't get kicked and scratched so much."

Make sure your tone and words do not imply that you no longer love your child. "I really can't stand it when you act like that" sounds final; "I don't like it when you try to pull cans from the store shelves," however, shows your child that it's one specific behavior—not the whole person—that you dislike.

10. Teach Empathy

It's rarely obvious to a 3-year-old why he should stop doing something he finds fun, like biting, hitting, or grabbing toys from other children. Teach him empathy instead: "When you bite or hit people, it hurts them"; "When you grab toys away from other kids, they feel sad because they still want to play with those toys." This helps your child see that his behavior directly affects other people and trains him to think about consequences first.

11. Give a Time-Out

If repeated reprimands, redirection, and loss of privileges haven't cured your child of her offending behavior, consider putting her in time-out for a minute per year of age. "This is an excellent discipline tool for kids who are doing the big-time no-nos," Dr. Karp explains.

Before imposing a time-out, put a serious look on your face and give a warning in a stern tone of voice ("I'm counting to three, and if you don't stop, you're going to time-out. One, two, THREE!"). If she doesn't listen, take her to the quiet and safe spot you've designated for time-outs, and set a timer. When it goes off, ask her to

apologize and give her a big hug to convey that you're not angry. "Nathaniel hated going to time-out for hitting his sister with the plastic sword, but I was clear about the consequences and stuck with it," says Angela Lampros. "After a few weeks, he learned his lesson." Indeed, toddlers don't like to be separated from their parents and toys, so eventually, the mere threat of a time-out should be enough to stop them in their tracks.

12. Talk Options

When you want your child to stop doing something, offer alternative ways for him to express his feelings: say, hitting a pillow or banging with a toy hammer. He needs to learn that while his emotions and impulses are acceptable, certain ways of expressing them are not. Also, encourage your child to think up his own options. Even 3-year-olds can learn to solve problems themselves. For instance, you could ask: "What do you think you could do to get Tiffany to share that toy with you?" The trick is to listen to their ideas with an open mind. Don't shoot down anything, but do talk about the consequences before a decision is made.

13. Reward Good Behavior

It's highly unlikely that your child will always do whatever you say. If that happened, you'd have to think about what might be wrong with her! Normal kids resist control, and they know when you're asking them to do something they don't want to do. They then feel justified in resisting you. In cases in which they do behave appropriately, a prize is like a spoonful of sugar: It helps the medicine go down.

Judicious use of special treats and prizes is just one more way to show your child you're aware and respectful of his feelings. This, more than anything,

gives credibility to your discipline demands.

14. Stay Positive

No matter how frustrated you feel about your child's misbehavior, don't vent about it in front of him. "If people heard their boss at work say, 'I don't know what to do with my employees. They run the company, and I feel powerless to do anything about it,' they'd lose respect for him and run the place even more," says Pearson. "It's the same thing when children hear their parents speak about them in a hopeless or negative

way. They won't have a good image of you as their boss, and they'll end up repeating the behavior."

Still, it's perfectly normal to feel exasperated from time to time. If you reach that point, turn to your spouse, your pediatrician, or a trusted friend for support and advice.

Ages & Stages

Effective discipline starts with understanding where your child falls on the developmental spectrum. Our guide: At 18 months your child is curious, fearless, impulsive, mobile, and clueless about the consequences of her actions—a recipe for trouble. "My image of an 18-month-old is a child who's running down the hall away from his mother but looking over his shoulder to see if she's there and then running some more," said Dr. Coleman.

"Though he's building a vocabulary and can follow simple instructions, he can't effectively communicate his needs or understand lengthy reprimands. He may bite or hit to register his displeasure or to get your attention. Consequences of misbehavior must be immediate. Indeed, if you wait even 10 minutes to react, he won't remember what he did wrong or tie his action to the consequence, says nurse practitioner Pearson.

At age 2 your child is using her developing motor skills to test limits, by running, jumping, throwing, and climbing. She's speaking a few words at a time, she becomes frustrated when she can't get her point across, and she's prone to tantrums. She's also self-centered and doesn't like to share. Consequences should be swift, as a 2-year-old is unable to grasp time. But since she still lacks impulse control, give her another chance soon after the incident, says Lerner of Zero to Three.

At age 3 your child is now a chatterbox; he's using language to argue his point of view. Since he loves to be with other children and has boundless energy, he may have a tough time playing quietly at home. "Taking a 3-

year-old to a gym or karate class will give him the social contact he craves and let him release energy," says Dr. Karp. "At this age, kids need that as much as they need affection and food." He also knows right from wrong, understands cause and effect, and retains information for several hours. Consequences can be delayed for maximum impact, and explanations can be more detailed. For example, if he hurls Cheerios at his sister, remind him about the no-food-throwing rule and explain that if he does it again, he won't get to watch Blues

Clues. If he continues to throw food, take it away from him. When he asks to watch TV, say, "Remember when

Mommy told you not to throw cereal and you did anyway? Well, the consequence is no Blues Clues today."

Chapter 7 Toddler timing and Developmental Milestones

Skills such as taking a first step, smiling for the first time, and waving "bye-bye" are called developmental milestones. Developmental milestones are things most children can do by a certain age. Children reach milestones in how they play, learn, speak, behave, and move (like crawling, walking, or jumping).

During the second year, toddlers are moving around more, and are aware of themselves and their surroundings. Their desire to explore new objects and people also is increasing. During this stage, toddlers will show greater independence; begin to show defiant behavior; recognize themselves in pictures or a mirror; and imitate the behavior of others, especially adults and older children. Toddlers also should be able to recognize the names of familiar people and objects, form simple phrases and sentences, and follow simple instructions and directions.

7.1 Positive Parenting Tips

Following are some of the things you, as a parent, can do to help your toddler during this time:

Mother reading to toddler

Read to your toddler daily.

Ask her to find objects for you or name body parts and objects.

Play matching games with your toddler, like shape sorting and simple puzzles. Encourage him to explore and try new things.

Help to develop your toddler's language by talking with her and adding to words she starts. For example, if your toddler says "baba", you can respond, "Yes, you are right—that is a bottle."

Encourage your child's growing independence by letting him help with dressing himself and feeding himself.

Respond to wanted behaviors more than you punish unwanted behaviors (use only very brief time outs). Always tell or show your child what she should do instead.

Encourage your toddler's curiosity and ability to recognize common objects by taking field trips together to the park or going on a bus ride.

7.2 Child Safety First

Because your child is moving around more, he will come across more dangers as well. Dangerous situations can happen quickly, so keep a close eye on your child. Here are a few tips to help keep your growing toddler safe:

Do NOT leave your toddler near or around water (for example, bathtubs, pools, ponds, lakes, whirlpools, or the ocean) without someone watching her. Fence off backyard pools. Drowning is the leading cause of injury and death among this age group.

Block off stairs with a small gate or fence. Lock doors to dangerous places such as the garage or basement.

Ensure that your home is toddler proof by placing plug covers on all unused electrical outlets.

Keep kitchen appliances, irons, and heaters out of reach of your toddler. Turn pot handles toward the back of the stove.

Keep sharp objects such as scissors, knives, and pens in a safe place.

Lock up medicines, household cleaners, and poisons.

Do NOT leave your toddler alone in any vehicle (that means a car, truck, or van) even

for a few moments.

Store any guns in a safe place out of his reach.

Keep your child's car seat rear-facing as long as possible. According to the National

Highway Traffic Safety Administration, it's the best way to keep her safe. Your child should remain in a rear-facing car seat until she reaches the top height or weight limit allowed by the car seat's manufacturer. Once your child outgrows the rear-facing car seat, she is ready to travel in a forward-facing car seat with a harness.

7.3 The right Healthy Bodies for your Kids

Give your child water and plain milk instead of sugary drinks. After the first year, when your nursing toddler is eating more and different solid foods, breast milk is still an ideal addition to his diet.

Your toddler might become a very picky and erratic eater. Toddlers need less food because they don't grow as fast. It's best not to battle with him over this. Offer a selection of healthy foods and let him choose what she wants. Keep trying new foods; it might take time for him to learn to like them.

Limit screen time and develop a media use plan for your family.external icon For children younger than 18 months of age, the AAP recommends that it's best if toddlers not use any screen media other than video chatting.

Your toddler will seem to be moving continually—running, kicking, climbing, or jumping. Let him be active—he's developing his coordination and becoming strong.

Make sure your child gets the recommended amount of sleep each night: For toddlers 1-2 years, 11–14 hours per 24 hours (including naps)

7.4 The proper height and Weight for your children

Baby growth charts for boys and girls are an important tool health providers use when it comes to comparing your child's growth to other kids her age. But for the average parent, they can be a little confusing to decipher.

To make it easier for you to get informed, we had experts breakdown the information you really want to

know about your child's physical development. Here's a simple look at average height and weight growth at every age:

7.5 Baby Height and Weight Growth

Birth to 4 Days Old

The average newborn is 19.5 inches long and weighs 7.25 pounds. Boys have a head circumference of about 13.5 inches and girls measure in at 13.3 inches, according to the National Center for Health Statistics.

A baby drops 5 to 10 percent of his total body weight in his first few days of life because of the fluid he loses through urine and stool, says Parents advisor Ari Brown, M.D., author of Baby 411.

5 Days to 3 Months

Babies gain about an ounce a day on average during this period, or half a pound per week, and they should be back to their birthweight by their second-week visit. Expect a growth surge around 3 weeks and then another one at 6 weeks.

3 Months to 6 Months

A baby should gain about half a pound every two weeks.

By 6 months, she should have doubled her birthweight.

7 Months to 12 Months

A child is still gaining about a pound a month. If you're nursing, your baby may not gain quite this much, or he may dip slightly from one percentile to another on the growth chart.

"At this point, babies may also burn more calories because they're starting to crawl or cruise," says Tanya Altmann, M.D., a Los Angeles pediatrician and author of Mommy Calls. Even so, by the time he reaches his first birthday, expect him to have grown 10 inches in length and tripled his birthweight and his head to have grown by about 4 inches.

Toddler Height and Weight Growth

Age 1

Toddlers will grow at a slower pace this year but will gain about a half a pound a month and will grow a total of about 4 or 5 inches in height.

Age 2

A kid will sprout about 3 more inches by the end of her third year and will have quadrupled her birthweight by gaining about 4 more pounds. By now, your pediatrician

will be able to make a fairly accurate prediction about her adult height.

7.6 Preschooler Height and Weight Growth (Ages 3-4)

A preschooler will grow about 3 inches and gain 4 pounds each year.

You may also find that your child starts to shed the baby fat from his face and looks lankier, since kids' limbs grow more by the time they are preschoolers, says Daniel

Rauch, M.D., associate professor of pediatrics at Mount Sinai School of Medicine, in New York City.

7.7 Kids Height and Weight Growth (Ages 5+)

Starting at 5 years old, kids will begin to grow about 2 inches and gain 4 pounds each year until puberty (usually between 8 and 13 for girls and 10 and 14 for boys). Girls often reach their full height about two years after their first period. Boys usually hit their adult height around age 17.

7.8 How to keep your little toddler always happy and joyful

What Makes a Child Happy?

We all want the same things for our kids. We want them to grow up to love and be loved, to follow their dreams, to find success. Mostly, though, we want them to be happy. But just how much control do we have over our children's happiness?

Happy toddlers don't just happen...they're molded by parents who care!

Bubbling giggles, chubby feet and colorful facial expressions all make-up a happy toddler!

It thrills my soul to see a content, obviously well-loved toddlers, explore their new world.

Their enthusiasm about daily life is contagious

But some toddlers don't enjoy the blessings of a home that's filled with encouraging words, bundles of hugs and wheelbarrels full of kisses. Instead, they face daily criticism and harshness.

Have you ever heard a mother or father yell "Shut-up!" to their toddler?

Unfortunately I have. I absolutely shutter and my teeth

clench when I hear those anger-filled words. Instead of tearing toddlers down, we should be encouraging them!

Our focus should be creating happy toddlers — not creating sad, frustrated, misunderstood toddlers! I'll admit it.

Sometimes it is crazy-easy to snap at toddler because you're trying to get other work done and they interrupt you once again.

Be present in your toddler's life. Don't push your munchkin away when you are answering an email. Instead take a few moments and address her needs or wants. Take time to play with your toddler every day. Make tents together, color pictures, go on walks, bake together, try these simple toddler activities or whatever your child enjoys doing — do it! My youngest child enjoys swinging on our large patio swing. I try to make a "date" with him everyday for this special time. We are making memories!

Set goals. Are you making dinner soon? Ask your toddler to help set the table. Do you clean your room in the morning? Ask your little one to help you make your bed. By giving toddlers responsibilities you are letting them know they have an important place

in the family. When a child successfully completes a goal, like chores, he begins to develop security and an "I can do it!" attitude.

It is my three-year-old son's task to open the door for visitors after they leave our home. He enjoys it so much! When he runs back to us, he always has an upbeat spirit and can't wait to help out in another area!

Establish boundaries. Definite boundaries help a child understand what is acceptable in your home and what is not. If she does not know the rules, she can become paranoid and insecure of messing up. Make your rules reasonable and make sure you stick to them! If rules are not enforced, they are worthless.

Examples of acceptable rules for toddlers: λ No whining or screaming.

λ Say "please" and "thank-you."

λ Pick up your toys after you play.

λ Do not open the refrigerator.

As your child obeys these rules, she will feel confident that she is able to obey "house ules."

By establishing clear boundaries, you are promoting even more security for your toddler!

Praise often. Criticism and negativity comes from

everywhere in the outside world. Create a haven in your home by praising your toddler for jobs well-done, good attitudes or any positive characteristics you observe. Praising a child always adds extra dashes of happiness to the soul! Use eye contact. When praising or correcting, get down on your toddler's eye level and speak one-on-one together. You are letting him know she is the focus of your thoughts and energy. When he asks for a drink, squat down and ask him if he want juice or milk. Take these special short conversations to interact with your child in order to build his confidence in your unbiased love.

Smile often. It's so easy to lose our smile when we're busy in daily tasks and life, isn't it? But a toddler finds much happiness in seeing a smile on mom's face. When a toddler sees that smile, the entire world seems like a peaceful, happy place...and the toddler knows that mom really does love and care for him! Our face speaks a thousand words!

Listen. Nothing says, "You don't really matter," like someone not listening to what you are saying. When your toddler gets excited about something and wants to show and tell you about this new discovery, really listen

and pay attention. Comment on their discovery. Don't just say, "Uh...yeah. That's neat. Now, go and play!" Your toddler knows when you're really listening and when you're just trying to shoo her away.

Laugh!. Go ahead, let your hair down and be super silly with your toddler. Sing silly songs with them, talk in funny voices — anything to get a smile or laugh from your kiddos. Adding some silliness and fun to your toddler's day is the perfect way to build them up!

Celebrate victories! Did your toddler finally get the potty-training deal?! :) Did your toddler learn to successfully and routinely nap?! Those are HUGE milestones and should be celebrated! Celebrate with just an ice cream cone, a trip to the park or some stickers! Keep it simple so it's always convenient to celebrate a new milestone in your munchkin's life.

If your toddler is struggling with napping successfully, we have an awesome super-loaded course for that! Yay for a toddler naps ,right?!

Chapter 8 Montessori toddler discipline techniques

"The first idea that the child must acquire, in order to be actively disciplined, is that of the difference between good and evil; and the task of the educator lies in seeing that the child does not confound good with immobility, and evil with activity, as often happens in the case of the old-time discipline." Maria Montessori

A Montessori approach to discipline consists of a delicate balance between freedom and discipline. Like any part of Montessori education, it requires respect for the child.

I'd like to share some Montessori articles that give more insight into Montessori discipline, which by nature is a form of gentle/positive discipline. As a parent, your greatest ally is the child's own desire to grow, to learn, to master her own emotions, and to develop her own character. By keeping calm and respecting your child and her desires, you can help her on her own quest for inner discipline. By setting clear expectations and supporting your child's active thought and reflection, you can support the sense of personal autonomy she is naturally seeking as she follows her

own unique path to physical, emotional, and intellectual independence.

8.1 Validate a child's emotions.

Of course, sometimes a child is going to want to take an action that is not permissible. A preschool-age child doesn't always understand why he is allowed to make some choices, but not others. Why can he choose what he has for dinner, but not when he has dinner? Why can he choose what to wear to school, but not whether he has to go to school in the first place? As an adult, you can help the child master himself in these frustrating moments by acknowledging his emotions. "You really wanted to wear your boots today! You are not in the mood for shoes! You're sad and mad about it." Be sure to allow your child time to experience the disappointment, and remember to save any reasoning or discussion until the initial emotion has run its course.

Montessori also encouraged teachers to talk with children about their behavior. To quote Dr. Montessori herself:

...if he shows a tendency to misbehaves, she will check him with earnest words...

Many people misinterpret the Montessori method to be a permissive method that allows children unlimited freedom. In reality, the freedom is within limits that are carefully enforced through guidance by the teacher. Common consequences in a Montessori classroom include:

λ Putting a material away that's not being used properly λ Cleaning up a mess or a spill

λ Staying close to the teacher

You can use these same consequences in your home.

Natural Consequences

When it comes to discipline, parents often feel the need to impose consequences and punishments on the child, rather than letting things run their course. However, this teaches your child to fear getting caught by a parent, teacher or authority figure rather than learning the natural consequences of their actions.

But, what are natural consequences?

In part, it's helping your child see what will happen as a result of their choices and actions, and letting it happen. Like what? For example, your child chooses to skip lunch. You allow them to skip lunch, but save their plate for later and when they ask for a snack, they can finish

their lunch. Or your child leaves toys out and doesn't want to clean up. You can explain that leaving toys on the floor is dangerous for others because they might step on them and the family needs a clean place to live. Then, you can clean up the toys together, ensuring your child helps. Rather than feeling threatened with punishment, your child learns to see how their actions affect themselves and others.

An easy way to implement this technique is by narrating what you see and helping your child predict the future. This also works well with aggressive behaviors like biting and hitting, and of course tantrums. You can say for example "I see you're angry. You want to hit me." However, in these cases, you may need to intervene to prevent children from getting hurt and say things like "I won't let you hurt your brother".

Montessori encouraged the use of control of error in materials and classroom activities. Natural consequences are the control of error of life. For example, Montessori encouraged the use of real glass dishes so that if children weren't careful or had an accident, the dishes would break. She believed this natural consequence was valuable for children to experience so that they could

change their behavior in the future.

8.2 Best way to make your kids grow faster

Most parents would love for their children to be tall and strong, as it has been widely regarded as a sign of good health. Parents usually go to great lengths to ensure that their children grow up healthily, and their height is treated as an indication of their overall health condition by most parts of the society.

Genes have the most say in determining the height of the child – however, it is not the only factor which influences it. Many external factors, like living conditions and a healthy diet, can influence the height of children quite a lot. Therefore, it is possible for parents to improve the chances of their children grow up to be tall and strong, through simple methods. Let us take a look at the top 10 ways to make your child grow taller.

8.3 How to Increase the Height of a Child

There are many ways a parent can influence the height of their child, and here's a list of the top ten ways.

1. A Balanced Diet

The most important aspect of how to increase your kid's height is to ensure that he gets proper nutrition. The food he consumes has to be healthy so that he grows up to be tall. A balanced diet has to include proteins, carbohydrates, fat and vitamins in the correct proportion – loading up on only one of these can have a detrimental effect. You must also ensure that the child keeps away from junk food most of the time – this includes food like burgers, aerated sweetened drinks and fried items in general. Lean proteins have to be had aplenty, along with leafy vegetables and items rich in minerals like calcium and potassium. Simple carbs like pizza and cakes have to be avoided for the most part. Zinc has been found to have a huge effect on the growth of the child, so zinc-rich foods like squash seeds and peanuts must also be added to their diet. A balanced diet not only provides the right nutrients to increase your child's height but it will also make him stronger in every sense.

2. Stretching Exercises

Stretching exercises, even if they are simple ones, can have a huge impact on the height of your child. Introducing your child to stretching exercises from a

young age will facilitate the process of height growth. Stretching helps elongate the spine and also improves the posture of your child at all times. The exercises can be simple ones. Make him stand on his toes with his back against the wall and stretch the muscles in his leg while reaching up simultaneously. Another simple exercise for stretching involves the child sitting on the floor with his legs wide apart, and reaching to touch the toes of both legs with his arms. Stretching exercises to grow taller

3. Hanging

Hanging has been recommended for decades now, for parents who want their children to be taller. Hanging from bars also helps the spine elongate, which is an important part of becoming taller. Apart from regular hanging, you can also encourage your child to do pull-ups and chin-ups. Both make the muscles of the arm and the back stronger and are great exercises to help him keep fit.

4. Swimming

Swimming is another healthy habit, one which helps your child stay active and enjoy it, too. Swimming is a full-body exercise, meaning that it works all the muscles

in the body to great effect. Swimming for a long time can help your child lose any extra fat present, making him healthier as a whole. The exercise involves a lot of stretching forward, which strengthens the spine and lays the groundwork for a tall, healthy body. Swimming is also a highly enjoyable activity- no child has ever said no to playing in the water!

5. Jogging

Jogging is an amazing exercise, not just for children- it has a range of benefits for grown-ups too. Jogging strengthens the bones in the leg and also increases the quantity of HGH, the growth hormone, which is required for any growth in the body. To make it even more fun, you can maybe join in with your child and make jogging be an activity you do together!

6. Sleep

The importance of sleep can never be stressed upon enough, not just for children – for adults, too. Skipping sleep occasionally does not affect the growth of your child in the long term- however, you have to ensure that the child gets a good 8 hours of sleep on most nights, in order for him to be taller and stronger. This is because the growth hormone in children, HGH, is released only when the child sleeps. This plays a direct role in making your child taller, so skipping sleep constantly is definitely a bad idea.

7. Posture

To increase your child's height, it is integral that he has a proper posture. Slumping or slouching can put unnecessary stress on the spine which can have many negative affects on the body. Additionally, poor posture can alter the shape of your child's spine which can compromise his growth. Make sure that your child practices good posture not only to increase his height but also to prevent any long term health issues. Remind him to sit and stand up straight every time you see him slouching.

There are many ways to make your child grow taller, but all of them work only when complemented by the other activities on the list. A good diet must be accompanied by regular exercise and sound sleep- else, you do not get what you want. Therefore, take care of your child the right way, and make him grow tall and strong.

8.4 How to keep your toddler busy and Happy at the same time

We all know that watching TV and playing video games isn't good for our kids. No parent is proud of how much time their kids spend in front of a screen but what are we supposed to do?

Sometimes, we just need to get things done. We need to clean the house or cook food or just take a few minutes for ourselves. It's hard to think of other things that could keep a kid distracted long enough to actually accomplish anything.

There are options, though. Sure, they take a bit more energy than just plopping a child in front of a screen, but encouraging your child to do something constructive just might be worth the extra effort.

We all know that watching TV and playing video games isn't good for our kids. No parent is proud of how much time their kids spend in front of a screen – but what are we supposed to do?

Sometimes, we just need to get things done. We need to clean the house or cook food or just take a few minutes for ourselves. It's hard to think of other things that could

keep a kid distracted long enough to actually accomplish anything. There are options, though. Sure, they take a bit more energy than just plopping a child in front of a screen, but encouraging your child to do something constructive just might be worth the extra effort.

Create a game box

Fill a box full of things your child can play with alone – things like coloring books, playing cards, or easy puzzles. When you need to keep your kids busy, give them the box. They might resist at first, but the more you do it, the more they'll accept "game box time" as part of their routine.

8.5 Have them make their own cartoon

Instead of watching cartoons, have your children make their own. Give them a piece of paper and some crayons, and ask them to draw you a hero and a bad guy. When they're done, let them come back and tell you their hero's story.

8.6 Let them help you

If you're cooking or cleaning, let your kids help. Give

them a job they can handle. For young kids, that might be stringing beans or setting the table. For older kids, that might be slicing vegetables, sweeping the house, or taking out the recycling.

8.7 Give them an important mission

Give your child a task, and make it a really big deal. Tell them they need to draw a picture for Dada, or that they need to make a block fort for Grandma. If they think it's an important job, they won't complain about working on it independently.

8.8 Generate an idea box

Brainstorm ideas with your children about what they can do to overcome boredom. Write down their suggestions, and put them in an empty box. Then, the next time they're bored, have them pick out one of their own suggestions. Given that it was their idea, they'll be more willing to actually do it.

8.9 Offer creative toys

Any toy that lets a child create is sure to keep them distracted for a long time. Invest in Legos, puzzles, and

Play-Dough. Not only will your child be able to play with them for hours, but they'll build up their spatial reasoning, too.

8.10 Design a treasure hunt

Hide something like a coin or a sticker somewhere in the house. Give your kids a clue, and let them run wild trying to find it. If you make it a bit tricky to find, you'll build up their resilience – and their ability to find things without begging for your help.

8.11 Let them play outside

Don't forget how your parents kept you busy. Just give your child a ball and a stick, and let them run wild. If you're worried about their safety, just keep them in sight of the window. They'll be fine.

8.12 Send them to a friend's house

Work out a deal with another parent on your street. When you need some time, send your kid over to play with their kid. To be fair, you'll have to let them send their kid over sometimes, too. When two kids play together, they keep themselves distracted.

8.13 Build a fort

Give your child a few pillows and a blanket, and challenge them to turn the couch into a fort. No child will turn down the chance to make a secret base – and they'll be much more likely to play independently once they're inside.

8.14 Make a sculpture

Give your child a few pipe cleaners and a piece of Styrofoam – or any other child-friendly items you might have on hand – and ask them to make a sculpture. Anything will do, but favorite heroes are a winning suggestion.

8.15 Listen to an audiobook

If your child's too young to read independently, pick up audio versions of their favorite books. Let them sit down and turn the pages while listening to a friendly voice read to them. Or, if you can't find a recording, use your phone to make one yourself.

Play with locks and bolts

Hand your child a lock and a key or a nut and bolt and let them play with it. Young kids, especially, will be

mesmerized by the act of unlocking something – and they'll develop their motor skills while they're at it. Give them a mixed bag, and see if they can figure out which lock goes with which key.

Conclusion

Congratulations! You have made it to the end and I want to personally thank you for trusting us with this very important stage in your child's life. I want to wish you all the luck so that you are successful in potty training. You have taken the necessary steps that many have not. You have taken the steps to getting the information so that you know what you need to do to be successful.

Remember, you want to be consistent. Consistency is one of the most important things that you can do right now for your child to help them be successful in potty training. If there is anything that you learn from us today, please let that be that consistency is crucial. Secondly is the 'push.' Every time your child sits on that toilet, make sure they are pushing. Once they push they can get up even if they have not done anything on the toilet, as long as they have pushed it is okay for them to get up. Remember that you are in charge. You are the parent and you have to set the stage. You are pulling the strings, so remember that as your child is trying to push the boundaries you have set. As a parent and as a human this process maybe frustrating. This process maybe tough and we understand that, and so

we're telling you to be parents and be human. You're going to be frustrated, you're going to be mad, and you might even yell a couple times.

But don't let that keep you from saying to yourself, "I'm not a good parent." You are human, it's going to happen, so you have to be yourself and do how you normally do things and be yourself and be happy and true to yourself. Most importantly, as we said, get some rest because you don't want to be stressed during this process. You want to have as much energy as possible. That not only will increase the chances for your child success, but help you maintain your sanity and increase your own success as well. We wish you good luck and lots of fun. Be strong!

Time-Saving Potty Training

The Golden Method Potty Train Your Little Boys and Girls in Less Then 3 Day the Stress-Free Guide You Are Waiting For

By

Serena White

Table of Contents

Introduction

Congratulations on purchasing <u>Potty Training in A Weekend</u>: *The Step-By-Step Guide to Potty Train Your Little Toddler in Less Than 3 Days. Perfect for Little Boys and Girls. Bonus Chapter with Tips for Careless Dads Included* and thank you for doing so.

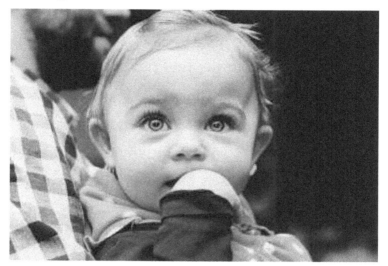

The following chapters will discuss the step-by-step instructions to potty train your child in just three days. Going beyond the bare minimum, this book covers not only just the physical steps that will need to be taken but also the mental preparation that will ensure that both you and your child are set up for success! This book will dispel the myths and misconceptions surrounding the potty training process and will outline how parents and caregivers can use psychology to make the potty training process more teamwork and less brute force. By

following the system outlined here, potty training will be a shared goal that both parents and/or caregivers and their children will want to achieve together! Not only will parents and caregivers benefit from learning how to create a spirit of teamwork during the process, but parents and caregivers will also learn how to handle the potty training outliers when potty training is not going as it should. Learning how to best support children in a variety of scenarios is an important part of potty training successfully and in a healthy manner.

To set the reader of this book up for success, it is important to begin with a strong knowledge base of the physiological and psychological processes behind potty training, or potty learning from the child's perspective. In other words, parents and caregivers need to know the physical and emotional processes at work during this period of time in order to best support their children through it. A brief note to the reader: Be prepared to hear some "potty talk" in this book! It is both necessary and healthy to be able to use accurate bathroom-related terminology during this process. Ultimately you will choose what terminology you use with your child, but for the purposes of this book it will be important to use bathroom-related language, so be prepared.

In addition to the real-life advice found throughout this book, there is also a bonus chapter that includes potty training tips and tricks from real-life dads for dads still in the trenches! All too often, books aimed at parents and caregivers forget that fathers are an important part of this team, and the unique relationship they have with their children can be utilized in specific endeavors like this for ultimate success for everyone.

There are plenty of books on this subject on the market, thanks again for choosing this one! Every effort was made to ensure it is full of as much useful information as possible, please enjoy it!

Chapter 1: In the Beginning

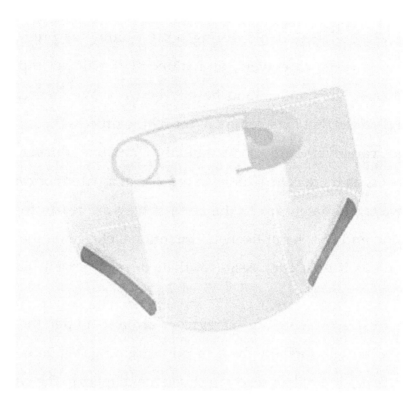

As you prepare yourself to begin the process of potty training with your child, there are techniques that you can use to prepare both yourself and your child to set yourselves up for ultimate success during this process! A significant part of this preparation will be the mental preparation because the mindset that both you and your child enter into this endeavor with will largely determine how quickly you are successful. The process of preparing yourself and your child mentally for the new journey you are undertaking is called priming, and it is going to play

a huge part in helping your potty training process run smoothly.To begin, you must prime yourself to approach potty training in a healthy and practical manner. Sadly, according to the American Academy of Pediatrics, the premier children's health governing body in the United States of America, the developmental experience that has the most potential for abuse of children is potty training and it is easy to imagine why. Frustrations are understandable during potty training as pressure is high for everyone: parents, caregivers, and trainees! It will be important that parents and caregivers understand how to best manage their expectations and any frustrations that may come up during the process.

Parents and caregivers are understandably anxious during the potty training process as there is truly only so much that a parent or caregiver can do. It is always ultimately up to the child if they are ready to ditch their diapers or not, and this is not likely an intentional choice on the part of the child as much as it is just the result of their developmental reality at that moment.

In addition to this, parents and caregivers are also under the additional burden of the actual work involved in potty training. While most parents and caregivers are more than ready to shuck the diapers to the curb for the additional ease and freedom of having a toilet-trained child, the reality is that there will be much more work coming down the pike before the child is fully potty trained. Before the child is fully potty trained, there will be plenty of accidents and additional laundry, as well as the extra mental and physical work of setting timers and organizing and developing a game plan that involves potty schedules and schematics for rewards and reinforcement!

Children feed off of this anxiety and pressure as they often recognize the importance of this monumental task being placed in front of them. This has the potential to create power struggles around toilet use, and nobody wants that! It is understandable that children will act out and push back against this pressure and anxiety, and this is what can lead to unacceptable and even dangerous uses of force from parents and caregivers as unnecessary and unproductive punishments intended to manipulate their children's behavior.Careful examination of the expectations that parents and caregivers hold over their children's capabilities as well as a solid game plan to complete the potty training process will help to set the parent and/or caregiver up for success with their children.Some of the expectations that parents and

caregivers hold around the potty training process are a result of myths and misconceptions around the practice that have been around for many, many years that we will cover now.

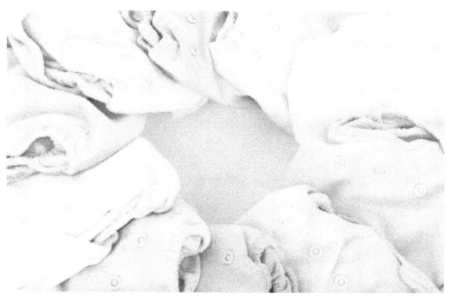

Myth #1

There is a magic potty training age that if a parent and/or caregiver begins, the child will be more successful in the potty training process.

Fact

Every child develops according to their own schedule! Potty training is not an exact science because every child will have their own distinctly unique timetable as to when their mind and body is ready will be ready to begin the process. There is no need to put extra pressure on

the process by ignoring the signs and signals your child is showing you as to whether or not they are ready to begin potty training just because the calendar says so! Most children potty train sometime between the ages of two and four, with outliers that begin younger than two and those that are still training beyond the age of four.

Myth #2

Potty training is something parents do to and for their children, not with their children.

Fact

This is as wrong as wrong can be! Potty training is not something that a parent and/or caregiver can do for their child, it is an interactive process that requires cooperation and teamwork from both parent and/or caregiver and child. You want your child to be your partner in this venture!

Myth #3

Your child is being willfully disobedient if they won't potty train according to your schedule and expectations.

Fact

While it could be true that your child is willfully pushing

potty training away, this does not necessarily mean that your child is being disobedient. As was discussed in the introduction, there are many reasons why you cannot force a child to potty train before they are ready. There are physical and mental processes that must be developed before a child can fully learn the skill of proper toilet use.

Myth #4

If you've already potty trained an older sibling using a specific method, then the younger siblings should also be able to train using that method.

Fact

Each child is their own unique and individualistic person with their own personal needs and capabilities. Each child develops in their own time and what may have worked for their older sibling (or their cousin, or neighbor, or playmate) may not necessarily work for them.

Myth #5

Once my child potty trains, there is no looking back!

Fact

This is a very common myth. It is not accurate however. Most children do go on to have accidents for some time after potty training. The window for becoming a potty pro is quite wide for small children, with some children having accidents up to a few years after they officially "potty train" and ditch their diapers. This is very normal. There is much to distract small children and it can be very easy to forget all about their bodily functions when they are learning so much every day about this dazzling new world all around them!

Myth #6

If we potty train our child to use the toilet during the day, we should potty train our child to stay dry throughout the night, too.

Fact

There are schools of thought regarding potty training that believe that potty training should be an "all or nothing" sort of experience, and this includes getting rid of any sort of diaper or pull-up type of training pants at nighttime. However, potty training at night is actually a completely different process than the process for potty

training during the day because a child's ability to stay dry throughout the night has less to do with learning proper toileting habits and bodily signals and more to do with night time hormones related to urine production and the degree to how heavily your child sleeps. Most doctors and urologists agree that nighttime bladder control is not an issue until the child is around seven years old.

As you can see, there are many myths and misconceptions surrounding the potty training experience that can set a parent and/or caregiver up for expectations that can't be met. Sometimes this is a result of failing to recognize what potty learning truly is for the child.For a child that has been diapered since birth, learning how to ditch their diapers requires a whole world of complexity that parents and caregivers often do not take the time to consider. For their tiny little bodies and minds, they have never had to pay much attention to their elimination habits. They've always just had their waste products exit their bodies when it needed to, without any real consideration or effort on their parts. To begin the potty training process, parents and caregivers must realize that they are essentially starting from scratch!The child must first learn to be aware of her body and its functions. This requires an awareness that what is consumed will need to then exit the body as a waste product eventually. For some children, this is a surprise! Taking the time to help teach them this connection is an important building block in the potty training process. They need to understand that the juice box they just drank will be ready to come out within the next hour or so, and this will be an important part of the methodology in Chapter 2 when you are introduced to the steps of the three-day potty training method.

In addition to being aware that what comes in must go out, children must then learn to be aware of what it feels like *before* they need the toilet. Again, they have never needed to be aware of the sensation of a full bladder in need of emptying in their life, their bodies have just released whenever they needed to without any help or awareness on the part of the child. This process of paying attention to the body and learning to associate the sensations of their body with the need to sit on the potty chair is often one of the most aggravating aspects of potty training for both the child and their parents and/or caregivers.

One way to facilitate your child's learning about their

bodily functions and the awareness of when they need to visit the restroom is to model this for them with your actions. This would include announcing to your child when you need to use the restroom and using descriptive language that they will understand. You will know your child best, but this could sound something like, "Oh, I think that glass of water I just drank is ready to come out! My bladder feels full, I need to pee/urinate/whatever terminology you choose," and you would say this while perhaps poking one finger into your lower abdomen over your bladder. Or perhaps you might say, "Oh, my stomach hurts a little bit down here, I need to poop/defecate/whatever terminology you choose," and you would also say this while motioning to your lower abdomen. The point here is to help your child learn where these parts of their body are so they can begin to associate these areas with making a trip to the potty. You are also teaching them the language they will need during their potty training experience.

The other crucial element here is in modeling the actual process for our children. Children are visual creatures, and they love to do what they see others doing! For most children, their primary caregivers and/or parents are their primary models of behavior and being allowed

to see a parent and/or caregiver sit on the toilet and go through the process themselves can give them a clear example of how they're supposed to do it. It is also important here to narrate the process for your little one, like this: "Okay, I have to pee now so I'm going to the potty. I'm going to pull my shorts down and sit here on the potty. Okay…. Now I just need to let my pee out! There it is, can you hear it? That's my pee going into the toilet! Alright, now I can grab a little bit of toilet paper, just like this, and wipe myself clean. Now I just need to toss it in the potty, pull my shorts back up, and flush! Ready to hear the toilet flush? Here it goes and WOO! Alright, now I get to wash my hands! I like this soap, it's blue. Pretty cool, right?" Notice in the narrative above that the parent and/or caregiver is not only narrating each part of the experience, but they are also making the entire experience sound like fun! Children will want to also be able to mimic this experience, especially aspects like flushing the toilet. The entire experience needs to be described like it is something that is a great part of growing up. This is a part of priming the experience for your child. If the experience is primed as something fun and attractive, your child will join you in this quest rather than resist you. In addition to this physical learning about the parts of your child's body and their awareness of them and what they do, there is a cognitive aspect that is required in potty training. Children must be able to not only feel the sensation of a full bladder or a bowel movement, but they must also be able to reason and rationalize with themselves to a certain extent. Young children often struggle with this part of the potty training process because it can be difficult for them to understand and engage in delayed gratification or time awareness. If a child is playing with their favorite toy in the living room, it won't matter too much if they feel the pressure of a full bladder and understand what that means if they don't have the cognitive skills yet to understand that they can set the toy down to go to the restroom and then come back for the toy again. For young children, they live in the moment, every moment. This cognitive awareness is one of the most crucial aspects of potty training and one of the reasons why so many of the "potty training tips and tricks" geared towards young toddlers do not work. A very young toddler simply will not have this cognitive awareness down enough to be able to make this choice, and this can lead to serious bladder and bodily issues when they are trained to hold their waste anyway. This is why pediatrician and urologist groups caution against enforcing any potty training protocol before a child is displaying at least the following signs of readiness: able to communicate their need to use the toilet either verbally or nonverbally, can physically get themselves to the restroom safely and efficiently by either walking or crawling, can dress and undress themselves to use the toilet, and can sit safely on a toilet seat unassisted. Enforcing a potty training program before a child is ready can result in urinary tract infections, kidney damage, constipation, and a lifetime of poor toileting habits.

Parents and caregivers can assess if their child is cognitively prepared to begin the potty training process by gauging how much interest and self-awareness the child has around all things potty related. Ask yourself the following questions to see if your little one is cognitively prepared for potty training!

- Does your child express interest in the toilet by following family members into the restroom or commenting on "going potty" when it is mentioned?

- Does your child express interest in "being a big kid" and want to do what older siblings and older children do?

- Does your child express when their diaper is soiled by pulling on the wet/dirty diaper, trying to remove it or even removing it themselves, and/or announcing that they need a diaper change?

If you answered yes to all three of these questions, then it is very likely that your child is cognitively prepared to begin the potty training process! Ask yourself the following questions to see if your little one is physically prepared for potty training!

- Is your child able to verbally and nonverbally express their physical needs, such as by asking for something to drink when thirsty or by stating they are cold and need a sweater?

- Is your child able to physically get themselves, without assistance, to the toilet and back by crawling or walking?

- Is your child able to dress and undress themselves efficiently enough to do so in the restroom largely unassisted?

- Is your child able to safely sit unassisted on a toilet or potty chair?

If you answered yes to all of these questions, then it is very likely that your child is physically prepared to begin the potty training process!

Once your child is demonstrating the cognitive and physical signs of readiness for potty training, then you can safely move on to the three-day potty training system! But first, a few words on the mental preparation moving forward.

You and your child will need to be a team in this endeavor. Not only is this necessary because one person cannot force another person to use a toilet (not safely and respectfully, anyway!) but it is also a matter of simple psychology.

Toddlers want to please their parents and caregivers- although it may not always seem like it! This perception happens because, for so much of those early childhood years, children have little to no bodily autonomy or control over where they go or what they do. This leaves them very few opportunities to assert their independence and capabilities in a healthy and constructive manner. This often translates then to what adults often view as being "petty" demands and tantrums, such as may occur over what color cup the child wants to drink out of or whether the child wants to put on their shoes or not.

Step back a moment and try to look at it from this tiny person's perspective for a moment: If you had no control

over what time you woke up in the morning, what you had available to eat, no capabilities to perform the majority of the tasks being performed around you (cooking, driving, talking on the phone, etc) and little to no choice over how you spend your days, wouldn't you also on occasion feel the need to make a choice of your own, on your own terms, no matter how trivial it may seem to others? This is the perspective of the small child, and the more that parents and caregivers can explore and understand this, the better they will be able to work with their child's psychology so that everyone can experience a win.

This is where the psychology behind team building comes in. Parents and caregivers don't need the potty training process to be any more difficult than what it already will be and should take all the help they can get! This includes the help of their small child, and it begins with how the child is approached with the process of potty training.

The child should never be made to feel as if potty training is an event that is coming up that they will be forced to be a part of, but rather should feel as if they are making the decision to begin potty training. This is easy enough to do for most children between the ages of

two and four because this age range is typically in the "I want to do it all by myself" mentality as they are looking to develop more of the autonomy and independence, they see being exercised by older people around them.

A note to parents and caregivers on how they speak to one another about the potty training process: Watch how you are wording your conversations within earshot of your small child. Keep in mind that children are almost always listening, even when they appear busy at play.

Comments that may not seem like much of a big deal can play into negative perspectives about the potty training process when heard by young ears that don't entirely understand what it all means. An example of this might sound something like, "We plan on <voice dropping conspiratorially> *potty training* this weekend," or "I just hope it's nothing like <insert name of child's playmate here> because their mom told me it was absolutely miserable! They spent months fighting it." This is even more of an issue for those comments that are made between parents and caregivers where there is visible negative body language such as head shaking, eye-rolling, or whispering behind hands. Children are more aware of these social cues than parents and

caregivers often assume, and this is not a good way to prime the potty training experience for your child! In the interest of setting up the experience of potty training as a shared goal and shared effort, look around for examples of meaningful models that your child may use for potty training. Is there an older sibling that they look up to? Is there maybe an older neighbor that is close to the family? Or perhaps a favorite cartoon character?

Remember, you want your child to *want* to potty train, otherwise, it will be you trying to *force* your child to complete this developmental process, and this rarely works. Think about other developmental leaps that children take such as crawling, walking, and even talking. Has any parent and/or caregiver ever succeeded in forcing a baby to crawl? Is there any physical way to force a baby to walk when they simply don't have the leg and core strength and coordination between their body parts? How about forcing a baby to walk that simply doesn't have any interest in it yet because they still prefer to crawl? No, of course not. Just as we encourage our children to learn to talk by modeling it for them and engaging with them verbally in a fun way, we can do the same with the developmental process of potty training. Keeping this in mind, enlist the help of

the meaningful models that you know your child will look up to and want to emulate. If it is an older sibling, ask the older sibling to join in on the modeling of bathroom behavior by both physically modeling the process and narrating in a fun and upbeat way. The older sibling can even say things like, "someday you will be able to do the potty just like me! Isn't that cool?"

If your child's meaningful model is a neighbor, you can ask the neighbor to announce before they have to run to the restroom, saying in an excited voice, "I have to go to the potty now, I'll be right back to keep playing with you in just a moment!" This would model both the process of making the decision to go to the toilet and also the idea that you can take a quick break from playing to go to the restroom and come right back to it.

If your child's meaningful model is a beloved cartoon character, then use that! There are a variety of ways that you can make this happen. There are many cartoon character toys that demonstrate the potty process and even sing cute little songs about going to the restroom, and they are available from major retailers; a quick google search will reveal what is available in that department.

There are also several cartoon episodes dedicated to

teaching children how to go to the potty, and these are available in many different streaming services such as Netflix, Hulu, Amazon Prime, and PBS Kids, to name a few. They are also largely available via a quick google search, so do take advantage of that!

One children's show that is renowned for its successful induction of children into the potty training experience is PBS Kids' Daniel Tiger's Neighborhood and their episode, "Daniel Goes to the Potty." This episode features the beloved main character, Daniel Tiger, learning to go sit on the potty. The song that Daniel sings every time he feels the urge to go to the potty is incredibly catchy and memorable and has been used successfully by many a parent and caregiver to remind a child that they need to go sit on the potty!

If you are a screen-free family and have no interest in using media to help during the potty training process, then feel free to be creative and make up your own potty training song for your little one to sing! The catchier, the better. Make it something fun and upbeat that your child and you enjoy singing every time they need to go sit on the potty. This is a part of keeping the experience fun and upbeat. It's amazing what our children will do in pursuit of light-hearted fun with their

parents and caregivers! To further prime the potty training experience for your child, you can determine how to best set up your restroom for your child. Many parents and caregivers choose to use an independent potty chair, which is the small, child-size potty that can be purchased at any major retailer/big box store or online. An advantage of this is the safety feature of it being their perfect size and situated firmly on the ground. There is also a feeling of pride in ownership that many children feel when they have their very own little potty, just for them to use. Some parents even take their children with them to the store to pick out their very own potty chair or give them stickers to decorate the potty chair and make it their own.

Another option is to purchase one of the seat modifiers that are also available through any major retailer and big box store or online that either attaches to the regular toilet seat or can be easily placed on top that makes the toilet seat a more child-friendly size. There are a few advantages to this, such as if bathroom space is limited and there is simply no room for another potty chair in the same room. Some children even prefer this option over the standalone child-size potty chair because they feel like more of a "big kid" with this option, and this

seems to be the case more often when there is an older sibling as the child's meaningful model. Another option that is similar to the seat modifier is to simply add a safety stool for the child so they can more easily get up on the regular toilet themselves. Often times this option can even be found with a hand-rail so they have something to keep their balance while climbing on and off. An advantage of this particular option is that it fulfills the same desire of the child to feel like a "big kid" in using the regular potty, and it also teaches them the necessary skills to navigate the regular-sized toilets they will find outside of the home. This can be very helpful for some children that may be uneasy about moving from the child-size options at home to the regular size toilets that they will find while using the restroom outside of the home.

Whatever potty option you choose, be sure to tailor it to your child and their needs. If you know that doing it "just like the big kids do" is going to be a big motivator, then perhaps it might be best to go with the options that modify the standard size toilet. If you know that your child doesn't like sitting on full-size chairs as well as smaller child-size chairs, then perhaps the child-size potty chair is best. If you know your child is always

excited to sit in regular-sized chairs to be "like a big kid" then using the regular toilet with a safety addition might be the right incentive for them.

Your shopping trip also needs to include some favorite beverage options for your child. This is important because you will need to have your child drinking plenty of fluids during the three-day potty training weekend. This is to ensure that your child is experiencing a full bladder and the sensations that come along with it as you teach your child to associate that sensation with the need to go sit on the toilet. Parents often opt for both regular favorites and "special" beverages that the child rarely gets so there will be no question as to if the child will be interested in drinking them. You know your child best, but fruit juices, lemonades, or any sort of sweet beverage is usually always a hit with any small child!

The next thing to gather in preparation for your three-day potty training process is the underwear that your child will be replacing their diapers with! Many children really get a kick out of picking out their "big kid" underwear, so take them shopping with you. This also plays into the pride of ownership psychology, in which you want your child to feel like they have some control here, too. Really have fun with this, talk it up at the store and make it exciting and fun to get to pick out underwear with their favorite characters, colors, and patterns on them. Remember, this is all a part of priming the experience for your child! Pro tip from a parent that has been there, done that: However, many pairs you think you need to start off with, double it. At the very least, double it! It is very likely that you will need them- and then some- during your potty training weekend extravaganza, so prep yourself well here!

Another important shopping trip that must take place before the three-day potty training process is the trip in which you procure the treats and rewards that you will use to keep your child associating potty use with celebration and reward. Parents and caregivers will know their children best, but whatever you do, diversify your treat and reward supplies!

Some common ideas for treats and rewards that are often used during the potty training process are small candies such as skittles, smarties, or M&Ms that allow for sweet, exciting treats to be doled out just a couple at a time. Stickers with favorite cartoon and storybook characters on them and little puzzle and workbook-style books that your child can interact with are always a big hit! Some parents and caregivers like to create a treasure box of sorts for the potty training experience that the child gets to pick out after they've had a successful trip to the potty, and this is often filled with a variety of sweet treats and small prize style toys. Dollar stores often provide a great value for this avenue, as you can buy many little exciting "treasures" for the child that won't break the bank! Anything that is new and different is typically enough to incentivize a child to want to participate in the potty training process so they can earn their rewards!

Some parents and caregivers choose to share the treasure box with the child the day before the potty training process kicks off by letting the child take a peek and know that tomorrow, they will get a chance to check it out and pick items out for themselves when they use the big-kid potty. This gives them an element of excitement to associate with the big day! Before the child heads off to bed the night before the potty training weekend, you can let them know that tomorrow you will be throwing away the diaper they are wearing and they will get to wear their big kid underwear and try the big kid potty! Let them know they will get to pick prizes out of the treasure box every time they pee or poop on their potty and that you will be right there with them to

celebrate with them. Make sure they hear that you are excited for the next day and you are confident that you guys will have a great day. Let your child drift off to sleep imagining the exciting things awaiting them the next day!In order to successfully utilize the Potty Training in A Weekend methodology, it is important to have a three-day long weekend devoted exclusively to the potty training process. This means that there need to be three days dedicated to the potty training process. No trips to the park, no running to the grocery store, no guests in the house to distract the parent and/or caregiver, and if you can swing it, siblings either 100% on board with helping be a part of this process or spending the long weekend out at a friend's house. The only thing you and your child should be doing over the course of this three-day weekend will be sharing this potty training experience!Parents and caregivers that have been there and done that during this process recommend ensuring that you have the laundry and other household chores caught up, including meal planning and prepping so that your mind can remain exclusively focused on the task at hand. There will be accidents- make sure you're not the cause of them because you were distracted taking care of some household chore! The Potty Training in A Weekend method has gained steadily in popularity over the course of the last decade, particularly in Western countries, with varying degrees of difference in each guide. The guide provided in this book is set up in such a way that you can learn about the many variances to this methodology and choose to adopt what you believe will work best for you and your little one. Just as every child is uniquely individual, so too is the home setup and the pattern of each individual household. View the guide here as a buffet of sorts: choose what you like and leave the rest. Your results will vary because every child is an individual, but Potty Training in A Weekend method, when approached in a focused and mindful manner on the part of the parent and/or caregiver, is guaranteed to provide a bedrock foundation for your child's potty training prowess. Your goal should not be a 100% accident-free, potty using a child at the end of this weekend, but rather a child who is well on their way to becoming one.Now that you have done the setup work to prime both yourself and your child to have the best mindset going into this process, you are ready to begin to delve into the step by step guide of potty training in a weekend.

Chapter 2: Potty Training in A Weekend

Day 1: Welcome to the Big Day!

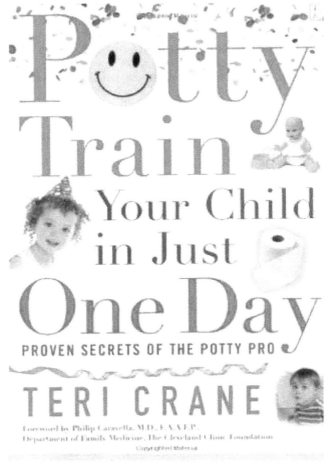

Wake up and get yourself set up immediately with timer reminders before you even wake your child up for the day. Most people choose to use their smartphone for this, but if you do not have a smartphone, then any clock, watch or another electronic device that has a timer and alarm capability will do! It is best if it is a timer that is portable and you can move around with you as you move around your home, but if you are using a stationary alarm such as a microwave or stovetop, then just be aware of keeping the volume down on other electronics and outside noise throughout the day so you can hear the alarm.

The alarm will cue you to each and every time that you will need to take your child to sit on the potty. This should be approached as an exciting, fun thing for the first day. Every time the alarm sounds, react as if you are thrilled to be hearing it. Your child will catch on to this and be happy to hear it, too.

Your first alarm needs to be set for exactly 15 minutes after your child gets set up for the day, so set that up as you go in to get your child out of bed. Building on what you began the day before, get your child out of bed in a fun and playful manner, reminding them of the exciting day you two have planned!

Keep your language here simple and direct so as not to confuse your child too much on what the day will contain. A sample script might sound something like this: "Today you get to start using the big kid potty just like <insert meaningful model here>! You get to wear big kid underwear and when you go big kid potty today, you'll get to pick a prize out of the treasure box! Let's

take off this soggy diaper and pick out some big kid underwear!" A lot of parents make a big production out of tossing this "last wet diaper" into the trash with their child and some even have the child toss it out and say something along the lines of "bye-bye diapers! I'm a big kid now!"

Let your child pick out their own underwear to wear and be sure that you comment on how fun it is to have underwear with their favorite character, pattern, or print on it. You can comment on the softness of the material or the colors found on it. At some point during putting the underwear on, remind your child that underwear is not a diaper and that it is not meant to be peed or pooped in. Be sure to include something along the lines of, "do you feel like such a big kid with your big kid underwear on?"

Regarding the type of clothing your child should wear during this intensive potty training weekend, the only real requirement is that it needs to be something that your child can easily remove to sit on the potty. Many parents choose to just use an underwear and t-shirt combo, but anything that slides down and then back up easily will work. You don't want anything complicated that requires buttoning, zipping, or even Velcro because

you don't want there to be any additional steps that your child will need to take to sit on the potty. You want to encourage as much independent movement as you can for your child around the potty. You want to help foster any associations between feeling capable and in control and use of the potty that you can.

Once you have gotten your child into their big kid underwear, it is time to begin the potty training process in earnest! Going into breakfast mode, allow your child to help you pick out what they would like for breakfast and announce to them they get to have a special drink since it is the morning, they begin their potty training process. Give them one of their favorite beverages that you have picked out from the store and encourage them to drink up. Let them know that they are going to fill their belly up with their special drink and then be able to go sit on the big-kid potty. Once your child begins to drink, set the alarm for 15 minutes. This will be the first time you put your child on the potty, and hopefully, the sugary drink will have done the trick. Let your child know that when the alarm goes off, they will be able to go in and sit on the big kid potty!

Once the first fifteen-minute alarm sounds, this will be your time to really play up the event. React to the alarm

as if it is the most exciting thing you have ever heard. Lead your child into the restroom (or depending on their excitement level, they can lead you!) and narrate the process as you go. "Alright! Here we go, off to your big kid potty. I'm so excited for you! This is great. Here we are, to the bathroom. Okay, can you pull your big kid underwear down, *all by yourself*? Awesome! Okay, now you can climb up to sit on your potty. Okay! Now let's check-in, see if there's any pee-pee in there that you can put in the potty! <Show your child how to gently poke and put pressure on their lower abdomen, above their bladder> Do you feel some pee-pee in there? Let's see if you can put it in the potty!!!"

The cycle of drinking a beverage and then heading to the restroom will be repeated throughout this first day, but one of the most important aspects of this ritual will be in the narrative that you provide during this process. You want to continue to provide the child with the physical cues of where they will be feeling the pressure of their bladder, so they will make the association between the sensations of a full bladder and going to sit on the toilet. For this first day, you will react with a celebration during every single visit to the potty. You want your child to experience a positive reinforcement of the association

that going to the potty equals fun and happiness. It is not necessary that your child actually uses the potty chair, today you are celebrating just making the trip! You will celebrate each and every time they sit.

Allow your child two to three minutes to sit each time. During this time, stay with them. You can read a book about using the potty, listen to or sing a song about using the potty, or watch one of the episodes about potty training available on various forms of media. Again, you are working to train your child to associate the sensations of a full bladder and pressure in their abdomen with the experience of sitting on the potty. Remember that you are building these connections from the ground up because they have never had to build them before! They have to move from mindless and passive elimination to conscious and mindful recognition and decision-making.

Again, this first day your child will get to pick a new treat from the treasure box each and every time they sit on the potty, regardless of if they go to the bathroom in the toilet or not. This first day is only for creating positive associations and teaching both toileting habits and how to be aware of their bodily sensations.

An Important Note About Accidents

Accidents will happen over the course of this weekend, especially on the first day. Do not be discouraged! Treat each accident as a neutral incident and keep your emotions level. Do not react as if it is a disappointment or a failure of any kind. A sample script for this scenario might be, "Ooops, it looks like you didn't make it to the big kid potty. Let's go take this wet/dirty underwear over here and get all cleaned up. Next time, we will try to make it to the potty in time!"

Keep your narrative around potty accidents neutral and matter of fact. This is going to be a normal and natural part of the process and your child will be learning that when they go to the bathroom in their big kid underwear, it is a different sensation than when they went to the bathroom in their absorbent diaper.

Your child is making lots of new connections this weekend, one connection that they do NOT need to make is one of shame, disappointment, and disgust surrounding the toilet learning process. Keep your reactions neutral and matter of fact and they will adopt that same reaction.

In order to minimize your own stress and anxiety over

accidents and the potential mess that can be made on furniture, some parents choose to either keep all activities for the day on the floor with a towel beneath the play space. Some parents even invest in some of the puppy pads that are available for dogs during crate training! These can even be put on furniture with regular bath towels over the top of them for both the added protection of your furniture against accidents and also for the extra comfort for your child! Be sure to do the same for the child's spot at the dining room table, as well. Mealtimes can sometimes be an extra tricky time for new potty learners to navigate paying attention to their bodily sensations and signals while enjoying their meals!Day one will proceed with the fifteen-minute intervals to sit on the toilet, keeping it an experience that the child wants to have with reading, singing, or media watching every time they sit on the toilet. Many catchy little jingles have been created surrounding potty use and they are helpful because children love catchy, rhyming, sing-songs phrases to begin with, and delivering helpful potty information is a way of reinforcing the potty experience for them. If you don't want to use one that has already been made, make up one for your family that you know your child will enjoy!During the course of this first day, any time your child does actually pee or poop in the toilet, be sure to make a giant fuss over this! You want your child to feel proud and accomplished and to always reinforce that experience of elimination on the toilet with celebration and acknowledgment. Going to bed that evening, be sure to tell your little one how very proud of them that you are, even if they didn't pee or poop in the potty a single time. Explain to them that because they will be asleep and unable to tell when they need to go potty, you will be putting special training pants on them (NOT their regular diapers, but something absorbent like a pull up) but will begin their awesome work on the potty again in the morning. This training takes a lot out of children, so be prepared for your kid to sleep like a log!

A Quick Note About Nighttime Potty Training

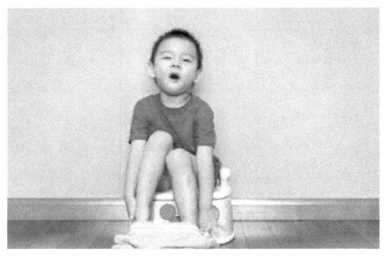

After a long day of visiting the restroom every fifteen minutes, you and your child will be exhausted! It can be tempting to introduce nighttime training at the same time but do be aware that this is not really something that can be trained but rather just something that a child outgrows and develops into. If your child often wakes up from their naps and their nightly sleep stretches dry, then nighttime training and trials with underwear have a great shot at success! However, it is very rare for a child to be dry during naps and nighttime sleep stretches but unable to control their bladder during the day. Typically, bladder awareness and potty training come before nighttime dryness.

By the age of six, approximately 85% of children will be able to stay dry, but children can continue to have nighttime accidents on occasion up until the age of 12 without it being considered an area of concern. Parents and caregivers know their children best and will be able to determine if nighttime toilet training should begin at the same time.

If you do choose to go this route, you will essentially continue the interval training as you do during the day, only with longer lengths in between. Instead of every fifteen minutes, you will set your alarm for every three

hours and will pick up your child (because they will be half-asleep!) and carry them in to sit on the toilet. Some parents use audio cues to help their children use the restroom in the middle of the night by turning on a nearby faucet. Once the child has gone to the potty, return them to their bed.

In order to decrease some of the time spent dealing with nighttime accidents, it will be important to use a waterproof mattress protector underneath the regular sheets. Some parents even choose to do additional layers of waterproof mattress protectors and sheets so that way when an accident occurs, the wet layers of sheets can be easily stripped away and there will be a dry layer already on the bed below. This can decrease nighttime sleep disruptions during the training process but do be aware that most nighttime potty training will be full of accidents if the child is not already mostly dry throughout the night. Again, this isn't really a training opportunity because nighttime bladder control has more to do with hormone production levels and those are produced on different timetables and have nothing to do with training.

Onward to Day Two!

Day two is much like day one, with one important difference. You will explain to your child that today, they will only be able to pick a treat out of the treasure box if they actually pee or poop in the potty. Do NOT mention accidents and be very careful about how you frame this information. You don't want your child to feel like they are being punished for having accidents, you want the emphasis to be on the reward for making it to the toilet!

Keep your spirits up and don't let up! This three-day potty training process is a *process,* not an event!

Day Three, Finally!

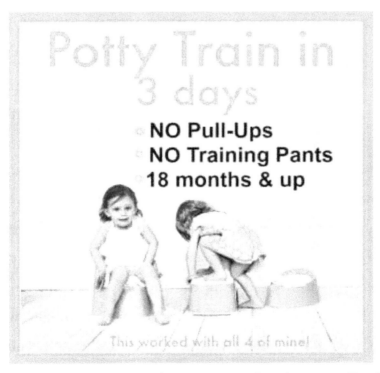

Day three is the day where big changes can often be seen. Explain to your child that today, you will be focusing on paying attention to your body and checking in. You will adjust your timer to half-hour increments, and rather than immediately traveling to the toilet to sit, you will instead encourage the "check-in."

"Let's stop and see if we need to go potty! <cue the gentle poking of the lower abdomen> Is there pee or poop in there that needs to come out? Should we go to try?" If it has been over an hour and your child still says they do not need the toilet and they have remained dry, encourage more drinking of fluids. Today is the day to really let your child figure out what these bodily sensations mean!

Chances are, your child is beginning to really connect the dots between what the feelings in their body mean and what they need to do about it. Day three is the day for them to really practice taking charge of this. You will still be checking in every half hour- and encouraging fluids- but you need to let them work out some of the cause and effect here, too.

Even if your child makes it to the toilet 100% on day 3, this does not mean that there will not be accidents moving forward! Small children are easily distracted and

will still require some cueing and reminding the adults in their life. This is normal!

Read on for the next chapter if you find you have a Potty Training Outlier!

Chapter 3: Potty Training Outliers

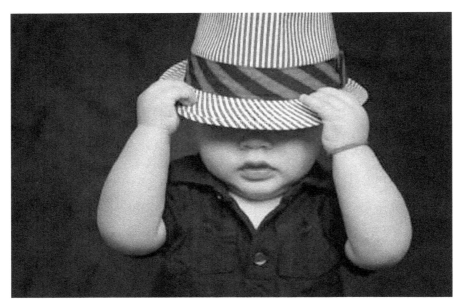

Some children will potty train earlier than their peers and some will potty train later. This is just a normal part of this developmental process! If you have a child that has potty trained earlier than two, then you still may have some potty work coming in the future.

Potty training regression is when a child who was fully potty trained for a significant period of time begins having accidents consistently. If this is the case, you need to look at potential reasons why such as if there is an emotional or traumatic event occurring that needs addressed (toilet accidents are often present during times of abuse) or if extra support is needed day to day. Consult with your medical professional to rule out medical reasons such as a urinary tract infection or

constipation.For children who are beyond the age of four and still not interested in the potty or successful after an extended period of consistent potty training efforts, then this is also a scenario in which you might want to check in with a medical professional to see if there are any health issues at play that are causing the delay.

There are children who will potty train early and those that will potty train much later, but outliers exist on both ends and are typically not a cause for concern. Children who are not successful with potty training programs between the ages of two and four can spontaneously train themselves seemingly overnight when they decide that they are ready. Again, there is very little that children are able to have complete control over in their lives and the toileting process can be one of those things that children for reasons that adults may not understand. This does not mean your child is being manipulative or trying to be difficult; it means that they are trying to meet their own needs in the best way they know-how and support during this time means more emotional support than physical force. Again, always speak to your child's doctor if you have any questions at all about health or well-being.

Bonus Chapter: Tips for Dads, From Dads

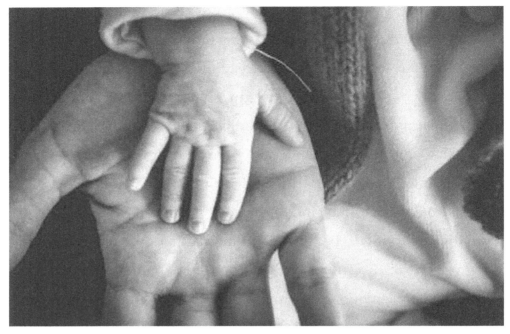

The relationship that a child has with their father is very unique and these are some tips and tricks that dads have shared with us:

"My little guy loves to do target practice in the toilet. I set him up with a few cheerios in the toilet and tell him to hit them as many times as he can and he is getting very good aim now!"

"My daughter loves to "show me how" so I like to pretend that I forgot how she uses the potty and she will walk me back to "show me how" and even sportscast the entire process!"

"I was worried about potty training and being away from home, but it's worked out really well so far. My son is really interested in all public restrooms, so anytime we end up at a store or restaurant, he immediately "has to go potty" which just means he wants to go see their restroom. It's working out though, not a single accident outside of the house!"

"Don't tell mom, but I still use Skittles. For pee on the potty, she gets two and for poop, she gets three. She never has an accident when I'm around."

"I let my daughter pick out a special foaming soap that she only gets to use after she's used the potty. It's sparkly blue and purple foam, so she makes sure that she makes it to the toilet so she can use some of her fancy "unicorn" soap!"

"I let my son pee in our backyard by our maple tree. We have a privacy fence so no one can see anything, and he LOVES it. I'm not sure what we will do in the winter, though…"

A lot of these dads have created playful ways to make the potty experience fun! Use your imagination to think of ways to do the same with your little one. Find ways to make this process tailored to you and your child and the things you like best.

Conclusion

Thank you for making it through to the end of **Potty Training in A Weekend:** *The Step-By-Step Guide to Potty Train Your Little Toddler in Less Than 3 Days. Perfect for Little Boys and Girls. Bonus Chapter with Tip for Careless Dads Included*, let's hope it was informative and able to provide you with all of the tools you need to achieve your goals in potty training your child.

Remember, potty training is a process and not an event. The three-day potty training method is intended to give your child a strong baseline knowledge of how to pay attention to and interpret the signals of their body and use the toilet properly. This doesn't mean that children will not have accidents as they go about their days, because children are easily distractible and after the fun of the three-day potty training method, going to sit on the potty won't seem quite as exciting as it did when they had a cheerleader on standby!

Continue to provide support for your child on their potty training journey and repeat the process as many times as you feel you need to. Remember that the potty training process requires a lot of your child: it is as much a cognitive process as it is a physical one. Be sure to tell your child each and every night that they are doing a

great job in learning how to use the big kid potty and that you are proud of all their hard work. Children that feel supported for their efforts, even when their efforts don't yield perfect results, will be far more likely to persist with determination than a child that is given the signals that because they did not do something perfectly that they have failed.

If you have been consistently potty training for an extended period of time with no results, consult with your child's doctor to rule out any possible medical issues. If none are present, then consider pausing the potty training process and revisiting it later. Keep your child in the loop of what is happening with as neutral language as you can. A sample script might sound like, "It seems like maybe you aren't quite ready to begin the big kid potty yet. We will try again in one month, okay?" It isn't a failure, just a standard part of the process involved in this major developmental leap! Kids that seem resistant at first may just need a little while longer to fully understand and grow comfortable with the process.

Besides, you can always be rest assured that everyone learns how to use the potty eventually. You will not be sending your child off to college in diapers, guaranteed!

Just as some kids walk later than others, some will potty train later, too. The day will come, believe it or not, you might even miss the days when your little one was in diapers.

Finally, if you found this book useful in any way, a review on Amazon is always appreciated!

Potty Training For Newborn Superheroes

Say "Bye Bye" to Diapers in 72 Hours. The Perfect Guide for Busy Parents That Love Their Baby Genius.

By

Serena white

Introduction

Parents play a key role in toilet training. Parents need to provide their child with direction, motivation, and reinforcement. They need to set aside time for and have patience with the toilet training process. Parents can encourage their child to be independent and allow their child to master each step at his or her own pace. WHEN TO BEGIN TOILET TRAINING YOUR CHILD There is no right age to toilet train a child the approximate time is between 15 months to 30 months.

Readiness to begin toilet training depends on the individual child. In general, starting before age 2 (24months) is not recommended. The readiness skills and physical development your child needs occur between age 18 months and 2.5 years.

Potty training might seem like a daunting task, but if your child is truly ready, there's not much to worry about. "Life goes on and one day your child will just do it," says Lisa Asta, M.D., a clinical professor of pediatrics at University of California, San Francisco, and spokesperson for the American Academy of Pediatrics. "When kids want to go on the potty, they will go on the potty. Sometimes that happens at 18 months,

sometimes it doesn't happen until close to age 4, but no healthy child will go into kindergarten in diapers." So don't stress — your child will ultimately get on the potty and do his thing, but you can help guide the process along. If you're ready to make diapers a thing of the past in your house, experts recommend following these seven easy steps.

Your child will show cues that he or she is developmentally ready. Signs of readiness include the fol-lowing:

Your child can imitate your behavior.

Your child begins to put things where they belong. Your child can demonstrate independence by saying "no.

Your child can express interest in toilet training (e g, following you to the bathroom).

Your child can walk and is ready to sit down.

Your child can indicate first when he is "going"(urinating or defecating) and then when he needs to "go." Your child is able to pull clothes up and down (on and off). Each child has his or her own style of behavior, which is called temperament. In planning your approach to toilet training, it is important to consider your child's temperament.Consider your child's moods and the time of day your

child is most approachable. Plan your approach based on when your child is most cooperative.

If your child is generally shy and withdrawn, he or she may need additional support and encouragement.

Work with your child's attention span. Plan for distractions that will keep him or her comfortable on the potty chair. All this and many more on how to get your kid on potty will be explain in this ebook.

Chapter 1 What is potty training?

Potty training is teaching your child to recognize their body signals for urinating and having a bowel movement. It also means teaching your child to use a potty chair or toilet correctly and at the appropriate times.

1.1 When should toilet training start?

Potty training should start when your child shows signs that he or she is ready. There is no right age to begin. If you try to toilet train before your child is ready, it can be a battle for both you and your child. The ability to control bowel and bladder muscles comes with proper growth and development.

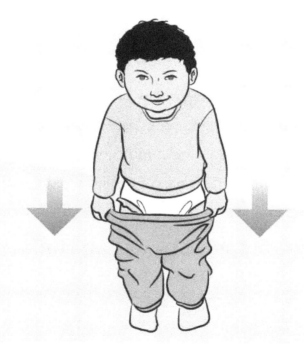

Children develop at different rates. A child younger than 12 months has no control over bladder or bowel movements. There is very little control between 12 to 18 months. Most children don't have bowel and bladder control until 24 to 30 months. The average age of toilet training is 27 months.

If you think your child is showing signs of being ready for toilet training, the first step is to decide whether you want to train using a potty or the toilet.

There are some advantages to using a potty – it's mobile and it's familiar, and some children find it less scary than a toilet. Try to find out your child's preference and go with that. Some parents encourage their child to use both the toilet and potty.

Second, make sure you have all the right equipment. For example, if your child is using the toilet you'll need a step for your child to stand on. You'll also need a smaller seat that fits securely inside the existing toilet seat, because some children get uneasy about falling in.

Third, it's best to plan toilet training for a time when you don't have any big changes coming up in your family life. Changes might include going on holiday, starting day care, having a new baby or moving house. It can be a good idea to plan toilet training for well before or after

these changes. Also, toilet training might go better if you and your child have a regular daily routine. This way, the new activity of using the toilet or potty can be slotted into your normal routine

1.2 General Knowledge of potty for children

You may (happily) have noticed that you're changing fewer diapers lately and your little one is usually staying dry during nap time. These, along with other signs, indicate that it's time to dive into the world of potty training. The key to potty training success is patience and an awareness that all tots reach this ever important milestone at their own pace. Different strategies work with different children, but these tips generally get the job done.

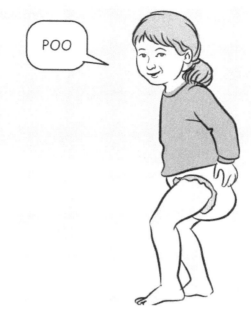

Since kids typically start potty training between 18 and 30 months, start talking about potty training occasionally around your child's first birthday to pique interest. Keep a few children's books about potty training lying around your house to read along with your child. And bring up the subject of the potty in conversation; saying things like, "I wonder if Elmo [or your child's favorite stuffed animal] needs to go potty" or "I have to go pee-pee. I'm headed to the potty." The idea is to raise awareness about going potty and make your child comfortable with the overall concept before he's ready to potty train.

If your child is staying dry for at least two hours during the day and is dry after naps, this could mean she's

ready to give the potty a shot. Before you head to the bathroom, know that she can follow simple instructions, like a request to walk to the bathroom, sit down, and remove her clothes. Also make sure she's interested in wearing big girl underwear. Then consider if she's aware when she's wet: If she cries, fusses, or shows other signs of obvious discomfort when her diaper is soiled and indicates through facial expression, posture, or language that it's time to use the toilet, then she's ready to start the process.

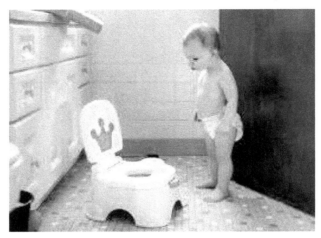

Some children are afraid of falling in the toilet or just hearing it flush, If your child is comfortable in the bathroom, try a potty seat that goes on top of your toilet to reduce the size of the bowl's opening. If not, you can buy a stand-alone potty chair and put it in the playroom or child's bedroom, where he'll become comfortable with

its presence over time. When he's ready to give it a try,

experts suggest you move it into the bathroom for repeated use, so you don't have to retrain your child down the road to transition from going potty in other rooms. Also get a stepstool — if he's using a potty seat, he'll need it to reach the toilet and also to give his feet support while he's pooping. "People can't empty their bowels and bladders completely unless their feet are pressing down on the floor.

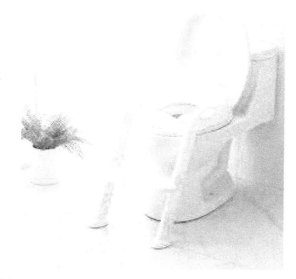

Even if your child seems ready, experts say to avoid potty training during transitional or stressful times. If you're moving, taking a vacation, adding a new baby to the family, or going through a divorce, postpone the potty training until about a month after the transitional time. Children trying to learn this new skill will do best if

they're relaxed and on a regular routine. You might prefer to get potty training over with as soon as

possible — maybe you're curious about the 3-day potty training trend. That's fine but do not always believe it, experts because you might find it frustrating not. "I often see parents who boast that they trained their 2-year-old in a weekend, and then say that the child has accidents four times a day, This is not the same as being potty trained. When kids are truly ready, they often will just start going on the potty on their own."

When you do decide it's time to start potty training, you'll want your child to go to the bathroom independently, day or night, so make sure she has transitioned out of the crib and into a big-kid bed. "Kids need access to a potty 24/7 if they're potty training so they can reach it on their own when they need it. Keep a well-lit path to the bathroom so your child feels safe and comfortable walking there during the night. Of course, if you think you're child isn't ready for a big-kid bed (or, let's face it, if you're not ready), there's no harm in keeping her in diapers at night for a while longer. Talk to your child's doctor about the best time to potty train your child; the

answer will range greatly by child, though most kids should be out of diapers during the day by age 3. When you're ready to start training, let your child sit on the potty fully clothed when you are in the bathroom to get a feel for the seat. Then create a schedule: "The key is having times throughout the day where you ritualize using the potty so it becomes more of a habit," Dr. Swanson says. You might want to have him sit on the potty every two hours, whether he has to go or not, including first thing in the morning, before you leave the house, and before naps and bedtime. Tell him to remove

his shorts or pants first, his underwear (or, if you're using them, training pants) next, and to sit on the toilet for a few minutes (allot more time, if you think he has to poop). Read him a book or play a game, like 20 Questions, to make the time pass in a fun way. Then, whether or not he actually goes potty, instruct him to flush and wash his hands. Of course, always praise him for trying.

It's not uncommon for a child who has been successfully using the potty for a few days to say he wants to go back to diapers. To avoid a power struggle or a situation where your child actually starts a pattern of withholding bowel movements, which can lead to constipation, you might agree to a brief break. But try to build in a plan to resume by asking your child, "Would you like to wear underwear right when you get up or wait until after lunch?"

When you're potty training, accidents are part of the process; some kids still have accidents through age 5 or 6, and many don't stay dry at night until that age (or even later). Never punish your child for wetting or soiling his pants; he's just learning and can't help it. In fact, doing so might only make your little one scared of using the potty, and that, in turn, will delay the whole

process even further. Instead, when your child uses the potty successfully, offer gentle praise and a small reward. You might want to use a sticker chart—your child receives a sticker every time he goes potty; after he's earned, say, three stickers, he gets a small prize. "However, don't go nuts!" Dr. Goldstein says. "A lot of toddlers will react to excessive praise as they react to punishment—by getting scared and avoiding doing the thing that they were excessively praised or punished for." In other words, stick with stickers, a trip to the local park, or even a surprise cup of hot cocoa—no need to go on a shopping spree to Toys 'R' Us. Less tangible rewards, like finally living up to the promise of "being a

big kid" are enough for some kids. Remind your child about the benefits of "being a big kid," like if he wore underwear, he would never have to stop playing in order to get his diaper changed.So this should result to setting children up with good hygiene habits that will last a lifetime, washing hands should be a routine from Day 1, along with flushing and wiping, regardless of whether your child actually went in the potty. The Centers for Disease Control and Prevention recommends wetting hands with cool or warm running water, lathering up with soap, and scrubbing for at least 20 seconds. Make

hand washing fun by buying colorful kid-friendly soaps, and make it last long enough by singing a favorite song, like "Happy Birthday to You" or the

"ABC Song," so the bubbles work their germ-fighting magic. Yes, toilet training can be stressful—for the parents, that is! But if you follow your child's lead, it won't be stressful for him.

1.3 Dealing with the emotions

In this step-by-step guide, we are going to take you through some really in-depth training and information that my I have put together over the years on potty training. Additionally, When it comes to potty training, most parents and most people think it begins with the child. The reality is that potty training is begins with you, the parent or the grandparent, the relative or the daycare worker.

When we get testimonials from our clients and they say, "Thank you, thank you, thank you," I always like to say, "No, thank you. You are the one that did the hard work, so you are the one that deserves the congratulations." With that being said, we are going to start with you, the parent, or you, the person who is going to be doing the training.

You must be prepared and know that this is going to be

a trying time, for some parents more than others. This can be a very stressful time because it tends to be a very stressful situation. What I want to make sure you understand is that nothing that is going on with your child with respect to potty training is your fault.

You have not done anything wrong. It may be as simple as the information you have received (or lack thereof). As an adult, what you know is that kids are not born knowing what to do and we are not born knowing how to be parents. Potty training, like many other lessons is something that is learned and you've taken the right steps in trying to acquire that information. So, the first step is to prepare yourself mentally for this project. Remember that your child has spent two or three years going to the bathroom in his or her diaper.

Now, you are going to ask them to do something that is completely out of the norm and, essentially erasing two or three years of habit. Saying that this is going to be a challenge may be an understatement as some children may battle and butt heads with you.

But being mentally prepared will help you in coping with the challenge itself. How do you get prepared? First, take your time, and get relaxed. Do whatever it takes to help you get into a relaxed state of mind. Its better if you can start the potty training process when have had a good amount of sleep. Being tired and trying to potty train makes it just that much more difficult.

You will also want to make sure your child is rested as well. This is just as stressful for them and being cranky while learning a new technique is not a good combination. Also, practice counting to 10 and then counting backwards from 10. This is a practice that you will find calms you down during periods of frustration in the process. In addition to being relaxed, you will need to ensure that you have a good support system. Talk with your husband or your wife or friends, and make sure that everyone is on board with what you are going to do so you are all heading in the same direction and can be a sounding board for each other.

This is critical because if there isn't a support system, the person doing the potty training will have a more difficult time and experience feelings of their own relating to the responsibility, frustration, and in some cases, failure (at least in the short run). If you are able to start this process on a weekend, it is highly suggested because you won't have the stress of work and you can have the dedicated focus needed to get this done right the first time. This can be applied to any period of time

when you can get yourself a good three days to focus and concentrate.

1.4 Using motivation for the training

A lot of products out there will tell you that to motivate your child, you need to go to the store and pick up a toy or something like that. And while that's good, I want to give you something even better when it comes to motivation. Here's the problem with giving them toys or

saying, "I'm taking your toys away," and actually taking the toy away and hiding it so that they don't see it. When children are between the ages of 2 and 5, out of sight, out of mind, the average attention span at that age is about 7 minutes. So, if you take the toy away it only takes 7 minutes before they never even realized they had a toy in the first place. So, that motivation does not go very far. What I like to do is instead is use fear of loss versus fear of gain. Now, let me explain the difference to you between fear of loss and fear of gain. Most people even as adults think about it today. We work harder to prevent ourselves from losing things than we do to gain things. Fear of loss is a bigger motivator than fear of gain. So if you are saying, "If you behave, you will get." or, "If you use the potty, you will

get."Although it can be a good thing for motivation, I think you can get a better response by saying, "If you don't use the potty, you will lose this." In other words, if they don't use the potty, they're going to lose something. Let me give you an example of one of the motivations we used to use with my youngest son. We had to "outsmart the fox" as I call it. I used to have to say something like, "Lorenzo, do you want to go to

McDonald's?" And he'd say, "Yes, let's go toMcDonald's." So, then I would say, "Okay, great. Go get your coat. Go get your shoes. Let's go to McDonalds." He'd go get his stuff and we'd open the front door and get ready to walk out. And then I would say, "Oh, you know what Lorenzo, let's use the bathroom before we go because you don't want to have an accident at Ronald McDonald's house." So, what did I do it at that point? Using a fear of loss, I defuse the potty. At that point, losing McDonalds was way more important to him than the toilet. So, he went without any issues at all. Now, granted, going to McDonald's means you have to spend money, but there are other ways that you can use the same methodology inside the house. For example, you can use their favorite cookie or their favorite snack. Let's say they like pudding. You might say, "Hey Lorenzo, do you want some pudding?" And the answer of course is going to be, "Yes." You then take the pudding, you put it on the table, you put the spoon in the bowl, you actually let them grab the spoon, get ready to take a bite and you say, "Wait a second, wait a second. Before you take that bite, let's go use the potty." At this point, the pudding and the reward are so real to the child that the potty is nothing. They'll use the potty just so they can come back and get that reward. You can do this with the toys as well.You can also do it with television. If it is a television program that they really like, then I would wait until the show is getting ready to start and I'd say, "Hey, let's go use the bathroom before we have an accident watching the show." If they said, "Oh the show is starting. I don't want to use the bathroom." Then, your answer is, "Well, we better go quickly if you want to see that show. Until we use the bathroom the show is not going to be on." Then, you can literally turn the television off. So, that is the way to motivate getting to the results. You don't want to use the same old, "I'm taking the toys away."

You hide the toys and they don't see the toys for months, and to them, they never existed in the first place.

1.5 How will I know my toddler is ready to be potty trained?

If your little one isn't developmentally ready for potty training, even the best toilet tactics will fall short. Wait for these surefire signs that your tot is set to get started: You're changing fewer diapers. Until they're around 20 months old, toddlers still pee frequently, but once they can stay dry for an hour or two, it's a sign that they're developing bladder control and are becoming physically ready for potty training.

Bowel movements become more regular. This makes it easier to pull out the potty in a pinch when it's time. Your little one is more vocal about going to the bathroom. When your child starts to broadcast peeing and pooping by verbalizing or showing you through his facial expressions, potty training is on the horizon.

Your child notices (and doesn't like) dirty diapers. Your little one may suddenly decide she doesn't want to hang out in her dirty diapers because they're gross. Yay! Your child is turning her nose up at stinky diapers just like you do and is ready to use the potty instead. Kids are generally not ready to potty train before the age of 2, and some children may wait until 3 1/2. It's important to

remember not to push your child before he's ready and to be patient. And remember that all kids are different. Your child is not developmentally lagging if he's far into his 3s before he gets the hang of potty training. Potty training success hinges on physical, developmental and behavioral milestones, not age. Many children show signs of being ready for potty training between ages 18 and 24 months. However, others might not be ready until they're 3 years old. There's no rush. If you start too early, it might take longer to train your child.

1.6 Is your child ready? Ask yourself:

λ Can your child walk to and sit on a toilet? λ Can your child pull down his or her pants and pull them up again? λ Can your child stay dry for up to two hours? λ Can your child understand and follow basic directions? λ Can your child communicate when he or she needs to go? λ Does your child seem interested in using the toilet or wearing "big-kid" underwear?

If you answered mostly yes, your child might be ready. If you answered mostly no, you might want to wait especially if your child is about to face a major change, such as a move or the arrival of a new sibling. Your readiness is important, too. Let your child's motivation,

instead of your eagerness, lead the process. Try not to equate potty training success or difficulty with your child's intelligence or stubbornness. Also, keep in mind that accidents are inevitable and punishment has no role in the process. Plan toilet training for when you or a caregiver can devote the time and energy to be consistent on a daily basis for a few months.

1.7 How to know when its time for a child with special need

While parents often complain of difficulty potty training their children, for most families, potty training is a fairly easy experience. Even when there are problems or children show signs of potty training resistance, usually, they will eventually become potty trained.

1.8 Signs of Potty Training Readiness in Children With Special Needs

However, this is not always the case for children with developmental delays or disabilities, such as autism, Down syndrome, mental retardation, cerebral palsy, etc. Children with special needs can be more difficult to potty train. Most children show signs of physical readiness to begin using the toilet as toddlers, usually between 18

months and 3 years of age 1, but not all children have the intellectual and/or psychological readiness to be potty trained at this age. It is more important to keep your child's developmental level, and not his chronological age in mind when you are considering starting potty training.Signs of intellectual and psychological readiness includes being able to follow simple instructions and being cooperative, being uncomfortable with dirty diapers and wanting them to be changed, recognizing when he has a full bladder or needs to have a bowel movement, being able to tell you when he needs to urinate or have a bowel movement, asking to use the potty chair or asking to wear regular underwear. Signs of physical readiness can include your being able to tell when your child is about to urinate or have a bowel movement by his facial expressions, posture or by what he says, staying dry for at least 2 hours at a time, and having regular bowel movements. It is also helpful if he can at least partially dress and undress himself.

1.9 Potty Training Challenges

Children with physical disabilities may also have problems with potty training that involves learning to get on the potty and getting undressed. A special potty chair and other adaptations may need to be made for these children.

Things to avoid when toilet training your child, and help prevent resistance, are beginning during a stressful time or period of change in the family (moving, new baby, etc.), pushing your child too fast, and punishing mistakes. Instead, you should treat accidents and mistakes lightly. Be sure to go at your child's pace and show strong encouragement and praise when he is successful. Since an important sign of readiness and a motivator to begin potty training involves being uncomfortable in a dirty diaper, if your child isn't bothered by a soiled or wet diaper, then you may need to change him into regular underwear or training pants during daytime training. Other children can continue to wear a diaper or pull-ups if they are bothered, and you know when they are dirty. Once you are ready to begin training, you can choose a potty chair. You can have your child decorate it with stickers and sit on it with his clothes on to watch TV, etc. to help him get used to it. Whenever your child shows signs of needing to urinate or have a bowel movement, you should take him to the potty chair and explain to him what you want him to do.

Make a consistent routine of having him go to the potty, pull down his clothes, sit on the potty, and after he is finished, pulling up his clothes and washing his hands. At first, you should only keep him seated for a few minutes at a time, don't insist and be prepared to delay training if he shows resistance. Until he is going in the potty, you can try to empty his dirty diapers into his potty chair to help demonstrate what you want him to do.

1.10 Tips for Potty Training Children With Developmental Delays

An important part of potty training children with special needs is using the potty frequently. This usually includes scheduled toileting as outlined in the book Toilet Training Without Tears by Dr. Charles E. Schaefer. This "assures that your child has frequent opportunities to use the toilet." Sitting on the potty should occur "at least once or twice every hour" and after you first ask, "Do you have to go potty?" Even if he says no, unless he is totally resistant, it is a good idea to take him to the potty anyway. If this routine is too demanding on your child, then you can take him to the potty less frequently. It can help to keep a chart or diary of when he regularly wets or soils himself so that you will know the best times

to have him sit on the potty and maximize your chances that he has to go. He is also most likely to go after meals and snacks and that is a good time to take him to the potty. Frequent visits during the times that he is likely to use the potty and fewer visits to the potty at other times of the day is another good alternative. Other good techniques include modeling, where you allow your child to see family members or other children using the

toilet, and using observational remarks. 4 This involves narrating what is happening and asking questions while potty training, such as "Did you just sit on the potty?" or "Did you just poop in the potty?" Even after he begins to use the potty, it is normal to have accidents and for him to regress or relapse at times and refuse to use the potty. Being fully potty trained, with your child recognizing when he has to go to the potty, physically goes to the bathroom and pulls down his pants, urinates or has a bowel movement in the potty, and dresses himself, can take time, sometimes up to three to six months. Having accidents or occasionally refusing to use the potty is normal and not considered resistance.

Early on in the training, resistance should be treated by just discontinuing training for a few weeks or a month and then trying again. In addition to a lot of praise and

encouragement when he uses or even just sits on the potty, material rewards can be a good motivator. This can include stickers that he can use to decorate his potty chair or a small toy, snack or treat. You can also consider using a reward chart and getting a special treat if he gets so many stickers on his chart.

You can also give treats or rewards for staying dry. It can help to check to make sure he hasn't had an accident between visits to the potty. If he is dry, then getting very excited and offering praise, encouragement, and maybe even a reward, can help to reinforce his not having accidents.

1.11 How to Use Positive Practice for Accidents

Another useful technique is positive practice for accidents. Dr. Schaefer describes this as what you should do when your child has an accident and wets or soils himself.

This technique involves firmly telling your child what he has done, taking him to the potty where he can clean and change himself (although you will likely need to help) and then having him practice using the potty. Dr. Schaefer recommends going through the usual steps of

using the potty at least five times, starting when "the child walks to the toilet, lowers his pants, briefly sits on the toilet (3 to 5 seconds), stands up, raises his pants, washes his hands, and then returns to the place where the accident occurred." Although you are trying to teach him the consequences of having an accident, this should not take the form of punishment.

1.12 When to Get Help for Special Needs Kids With Potty Training Difficulties

While it may take some time and require a lot of patience, many children with special needs can be potty trained by the age of 3 to 5 years. 3 If you continue to have problems or your child is very resistant, then consider getting professional help.

In addition to your pediatrician, you might get help from an occupational therapist, especially if your child has some motor delays causing the potty training difficulty, a child psychologist, especially if your child is simply resistant to potty training and a developmental pediatrician

1.13 When it's time to begin potty training:

Choose your words. Decide which words you're going to

use for your child's bodily fluids. Avoid negative words, such as dirty or stinky. Prepare the equipment. Place a potty chair in the bathroom or, initially, wherever your child is spending most of his or her time. Encourage your child to sit on the potty chair in clothes to start out. Make sure your child's feet rest on the floor or a stool. Use simple, positive terms to talk about the toilet. You might dump the contents of a dirty diaper into the potty chair and toilet to show their purpose. Have your child flush the toilet. Schedule potty breaks. Have your child sit on the potty chair or toilet without a diaper for a few minutes at two-hour intervals, as well as first thing in the morning and right after naps. For boys, it's often best to master urination sitting down, and then move to standing up after bowel training is complete. Stay with your child and read a book together or play with a toy while he or she sits. Allow your child to get up if he or she wants. Even if your child simply sits there, offer praise for trying — and remind your child that he or she can try again later. Bring the potty chair with you when you're away from home with your child.

Get there

Fast! When you notice signs that your child might need to use the toilet such as squirming, squatting or holding

the genital area respond quickly. Help your child become familiar with these signals, stop what he or she is doing, and head to the toilet. Praise your child for telling you when he or she has to go. Keep your child in loose, easy-to-remove clothing.

Explain hygiene. Teach girls to spread their legs and wipe carefully from front to back to prevent bringing germs from the rectum to the vagina or bladder. Make sure your child washes his or her hands afterward. Ditch the diapers. After a couple of weeks of successful potty breaks and remaining dry during the day, your child might be ready to trade diapers for training pants or underwear. Celebrate the transition. Let your child return to diapers if he or she is unable to remain dry. Consider using a sticker or star chart for positive reinforcement.

Chapter 2 Getting started with toilet training

The following tips may help you get started with potty training:

If there are siblings, ask them to let the younger child see you praising them for using the toilet.

It's best to use a potty chair on the floor rather than putting the child on the toilet for training. The potty chair is more secure for most children. Their feet reach the floor and there is no fear of falling off. If you decide to use a seat that goes over the toilet, use a footrest for your child's feet. Let your child play with the potty. They can sit on it with clothes on and later with diapers off. This way they can get used to it. Never strap your child to the potty chair. Children should be free to get off the potty when they want. Your child should not sit on the potty for more than 5 minutes. Sometimes children have a bowel movement just after the diaper is back on because the diaper feels normal. Don't get upset or punish your child. You can try taking the dirty diaper off and putting the bowel movement in the potty with your child watching you. This may help your child understand that you want the bowel movement in the potty.

If your child has a normal time for bowel movements (such as after a meal), take your child to the potty at

that time of day. If your child acts a certain way when having a bowel movement (such as stooping, getting quiet, going to the corner), try taking your child to potty when he or she shows it is time.

If your child wants to sit on the potty, stay next to your child and talk or read a book. It's good to use words for what your child is doing (such as potty, pee, or poop). Then your child learns the words to tell you. Remember that other people will hear these words. Don't use words that will offend, confuse, or embarrass others or your child. Don't use words such as dirty, naughty, or stinky to describe bowel movements and urine. Use a simple, matter-of-fact tone.

If your child gets off the potty before urinating or passing a bowel movement, be calm. Don't scold. Try again later. If your child successfully uses the potty, give plenty of praise such as a smile, clap, or hug. Children learn from copying adults and other children. It may help if your child sits on the potty chair while you are using the toilet.

Children often follow parents into the bathroom. This may be one time they are willing to use the potty. Start out by teaching boys to sit down for passing urine. At first, it is hard to control starting and stopping while standing. Boys will try to stand to urinate when they see other boys standing.

Some children learn by pretending to teach a doll to go potty. Get a doll that has a hole in its mouth and diaper area. Your child can feed and "teach" the doll to pull down its pants and use the potty. Make this teaching fun for your child.

Make going to the potty a part of your child's daily routine. Do this first thing in the morning, after meals and naps, and before going to bed.

2.1 After training is started

The following tips may help you once the training is started: Once your child starts using the potty and can tell you they need to go, taking them to the potty at regular times or reminding them too many times to go to the potty is not necessary.

You may want to start using training pants. Wearing underpants is a sign of growing up, and most children like being a "big girl or big boy." Wearing diapers once potty training has been started may be confusing for your child. If your child has an accident while in training pants, don't punish. Be calm and clean up without making a fuss about it.

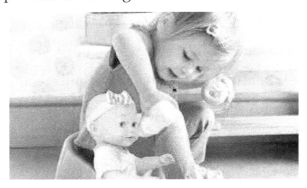

Keep praising or rewarding your child every step of the way. Do this for pulling down pants, for sitting on the potty, and for using the potty. If you show that you are pleased when your child urinates or has bowel movements in the potty, your child is more likely to use the potty next time. As children get older, they can learn to wipe themselves and wash hands after going to the bathroom. Girls should be taught to wipe from front to back so that germs from bowel movement are not wiped into the urinary area. Remember that every child is different and learns toilet training at his or her own pace. If things are going poorly with toilet training, it's better to put diapers back on for a few weeks and try again later. In general, have a calm, unhurried approach to toilet training. Most children have bowel control and daytime urine control by age 3 or 4. Soiling or daytime wetting after this age should be discussed with your child's healthcare provider. Nighttime control usually

comes much later than daytime control. Complete nighttime control may not happen until your child is 4 or 5 years old, or even older. If your child is age 5 or older and does not stay dry at night, you should discuss this with your child's healthcare provider.

Even when children are toilet trained, they may have some normal accidents (when excited or playing a lot), or setbacks due to illness or emotional situations. If accidents or setbacks happen, be patient. Examples of emotional situations include moving to a new house, a family illness or death, or a new baby in the house. In fact, if you know an emotional situation is going to be happening soon, don't start toilet training. Wait for a calmer time.

2.2 Potty Training Chairs

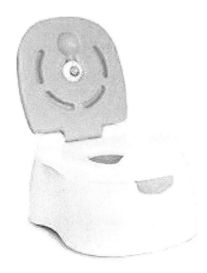

Many parents ask, "Do I need a potty training chair to be successful in potty training?" The answer to that question is "yes" and "no". For even our own kids, I used potty training chairs for two and no potty training chairs for our third child.

Now, he was an advanced child. He was doing things that the other kids never did so he never even wanted to use the potty chair. Even today as a 6-year-old in kindergarten, he doesn't like doing things that the other kindergarten kids like to do.

He calls them "babies." But I will tell you this: having a potty training chair does several things for your child. First of all, it gives them flexibility. When they have a potty training chair, more than likely it is mobile, which means that it can be placed anywhere around the house including the TV room or the game room.

This increases the success rate of your child using the potty. The rationale? Well, as you might already know, if you're in any other room than the bathroom when you see kids doing a pee-pee dance or you realize that they've got to go, it's already too late. That pee or the bowel movement is almost on its way out the door. But with a mobile potty chair, you can place it near their activities and in different rooms, so when the child feels the need to go, they don't have to rush all the way to the bathroom. They can simply get up and go in the vicinity of wherever they are.

Not only that, the act of running and holding for child that young is a very challenging thing. So trying to run to the bathroom from outside is almost asking for trouble. What you want to do instead is make sure that if you are going to use a potty chair, is that it's available and near. A potty chair is also great especially if you have a 2-story house and the bathroom is upstairs. You can then put the potty chair downstairs and cut out that climb. And the way potty chairs are designed today, they're colorful, they are cute and kids love them. It just is a fun thing for them and they always get a sense of pride because it's their chair and nobody else's. What we used to do is put the potty chair in a laundry room because there was a door there. My son would be able to close the door so we couldn't see him and he would have his privacy.

2.3 Starting the process

There are three different times that you can start the training process. Early when the child is 2 or younger Middle between the ages of 2 and 3, maybe 3 1/2 Later

between 3, 3 1/2 and older The optimal time for me is the age of 2. And, I mean the day they turned 2 is when we normally like to start with potty training. With all the years that I have been in day care and all the children that I have potty trained, I started every single one the day they turned 2. Even our own kids, we started them at the age of 2.

Now, starting at a later time is okay and that is the case with most parents. But I want to explain to you the difference between starting at the age of 2 and starting later. The key difference in starting at the age of 2 is that the child hasn't developed all of their social skills yet and their ability to go out and have fun is limited.

At the age of 2 and somewhere between 2 and 3 is when they find their own voice. (You've heard of the terrible '2s'!?) They find their own voice and they find their own spirit and that's when they decide that they want to start doing their own thing. When you start earlier in the potty training process it is easier to get them to follow directions and it is just easier to get them to do what you want them to do versus them wanting to do what they want to do. Now, girls can start even earlier than 2. Usually girls can start about 3 or 4 months before their 2nd birthday. Girls, as we know, even later on in life, are

a lot smarter than boys and men, and I will be the first to admit that. The earliest we've seen was a little girl in my class that was only 15 months that was potty training and doing a fantastic job. But some kids can start as early as 18 or 19 months, including boys. So, potty training earlier is great because it gives you the ability to control the process versus them being in control. When you start at that middle time frame, which is between 2 and 3 or 2 1/2 to 3 or later than that, what happens is that child goes more into the independent stage.

That's where they're able to start making to some of their decisions which happens to often include the word "no". And thus what happens as a parent is you're not only dealing with potty training but you're also dealing with behavior as the result of a child that is looking to find their self and their voice. Starting late doesn't mean you did anything wrong, and it doesn't mean that you're not going to potty train.; All it means is that it's going to be a little bit more challenging and a little bit more work. And that's okay but it just means that it's going to take a little bit more time to get the child potty trained.

Now, the other thing that you want to realize is the later you start, the more years of behavior modification you're

trying to reverse and that can account for some of that difficulty. In other words, when you start the potty training at the age of 2, you only have 2 years of pooping in their diaper or potty in the diaper to reverse. Whereas the later you start, let's say at the age of 3, you've got 3, 3 1/2 years of pooping in their diaper or the potty behavior that you have to reverse. So, it's a

very big difference starting earlier than later because it's a lot more habit that has to be broken and a new habit learned. To drive this point home, just think about how hard it is to change a behavior or a habit in yourself. If you think it's hard for yourself, think about a child that doesn't have the same cognitive ability that you have. Trying to get rid of that behavior as early as possible is better because it's less work for the child. We want to keep in mind how hard that child actually has to work to do this. The key also is that we're looking at doing this in just 3 days through consistency. So, reversing years of behavior in just 3 days is even that much more challenging the older they are.

2.4 Pre-potty training

Pre-potty training is getting the child ready for what is about to come if you really want to potty train him

within 3 days, or what it is about to happen. In other words, you set a time when you're going to start potty training. It's now February and you want to start potty-training in September or something to that effect. Before September comes around, there are things that you can do that will make the potty training process not only easier for yourself, but also easier for the child.

The first thing you want to do is sit your child down and explain what is expected of them. Sitting down is an important component of this.

You want to sit next to them or across from them and in a very loving and caring tone, you want to say, "I am going to explain potty training to you." And you want to say, "Potty training is when you go the bathroom (tinkle, pee or poopy) in the potty." Now in terms of the words that you use, you want to be consistent. If you call it "tinkle" then you want to continue using the word "tinkle". If you call it "poopy", then continue using the word "poopy".

As a young child, too many words are going to confuse them, so staying consistent with your terminology will help you enforce the concept and they will know exactly what it means. You want to be strong and direct. By that I mean using words like, "Mommy is going to have you potty trained, and here's what you have to do for Mommy...poopy, tinkle, etc." Or, "When you have to go potty, you have to let Mommy know, and you have to sit on the toilet and then you go potty". Then, you physically walk them to the toilet and show them and say, "Here is where you go tinkle and poopy." This isn't being strict; it's being direct so that they know that you are in charge, and what is expected of them.

If you don't take it direct tone, kids are extremely smart. They can sense a lack of control and they might not follow your directions as well if you say, "Mommy would like" or, "It would be nice if you"".

Take them to the bathroom and get them use to seeing you in the bathroom. Let them sit down on the toilet. Let them get used to having the toilet touch their skin as well. Many parents don't realize this, but many children have a fear of being on the toilet as opposed to just being hard to potty train. So this might help them get over that fear so when the potty training begins, you don't have to battle two things.

One thing is to start using less absorbent diapers. Today, the diapers are so absorbent the child doesn't even realize that they are wet. And most kids do not like the feeling of being wet. So when they have on a less

absorbent diaper, it helps them realize the act of letting go and releasing 'number 1'. But the wet feeling also starts to psychologically or subconsciously say to them,

"When I get this feeling of letting go, I start to feel wet too, and I don't like that." You will also want to make sure that you change them frequently when they wet their diapers. This helps them get used to the feeling of being dry and staying dry. It also reinforces the feelings they have once they wet again. It is also highly encouraged that you actually consider taking your child out of diapers while they are awake a couple of months prior to the actual potty training process. So, during nap time, you will use diapers, but during their waking hours, you will want them in big boy and big girl underwear. You will also want to make sure that this whole pre-potty training process is a loving experience because you want it to subconsciously erase some of the other negative connotations and fears that your child may have. It's important that you understand pre potty training is not a necessary step. It gives you an advantage if you are starting the potty training process early, but if you are like most parents, then you might have missed the stage or the time when you could have pre-potty trained. You can still pre-potty train if you

prefer, no matter at which stage you are, but it's usually better if you can start as early as possible. Knowing what we know and from our customers, however, most parents usually has missed this stage to the degree that they can get the most effectiveness out of it.

Chapter 3 Four stages of Potty training

In this section, I am going to teach you four stages to potty training. What you will notice and then appreciate is that these four stages can be applied to almost any other learned or practiced behavior which you are trying to alter or change.

3.1 The four stages of any behavior modification model include:

Unconscious incompetence

Conscious incompetence

Conscious competence

Unconscious competence

And now, I'll break these down to help you understand what they are and what you need to focus on during each one of these different stages.

Stage One: Unconscious Incompetence:

This is the "I do not know" stage, where your child's mind is thinking, "I do not know that going to the bathroom in my diaper is a wrong thing". In other words, the child has no idea that what they are doing is something they should not be doing. During stage one,

when they don't know the difference, this is when it becomes your responsibility to educate them and get

them to understand what they are doing is not something they should be doing.

This is where you are teaching the child that they do not need to be going to the bathroom in their diaper.

Stage Two: Conscious Incompetence

At this stage, the child has reached an understanding where they know what they're doing is something they should not do, but have no idea how to correct it. During stage two you are taking it to that next level where you are reinforcing the positive behavior by showing them where they are supposed to go to the bathroom—in the potty. So, now you're teaching the child where to go, how to go, and what to do.

Stage Three: Conscious Incompetence

Here, the child knows what they are doing is something they shouldn't be doing, they know what to do about it, but they are also not that great at it. They have to think about it. That is because the process is now occurring on the conscious level. It is during stage three that the child starts to understand on their own and they start to show you the signs that they can do this on their own as well.

This is when you should be getting to the point of not having accidents anymore. Now, this is an area where most parents go wrong in that they get to stage three

and they say, "My child is potty trained, there is nothing else that I have to do." In reality, this is where the real potty training begins. This is where you really want to be consistent to ensure they reach stage four and can consistently go to the potty by themselves. So, when you get to stage three, you have to make sure that you continue with consistency.

Stage Four: Unconscious Competence

And this is the fun stage. This is when the child gets to where they need to should know what they're doing and they don't have to think about it any longer. It is at stage four that your child can be officially considered 'potty trained.' Let's take a quick example to make sure the concept sinks in: If you are in stage three, you're not showing the child where to go potty anymore because they know where to go. What you're doing is being consistent with them going to the potty on a regular basis. During stage two you're not so much worried about consistency yet, you are more focused on helping them know where to go. Hopefully this description has given you a better understanding of how each stage develops and, better yet, what your actions need to be during each stage.

3.2 Potty Training as a young Mother

As a young mum who have no much experience about potty training; one of the best thing you can do to help your kid is to be a positive potty model. When you go to the bathroom, use it as an opportunity to talk your child through the process. Use words he or she can say, like pee, poop, and potty. If you plan to start your child on a potty seat, put it in the bathroom so it becomes familiar. Make it a fun place your child wants to sit, with or without the diaper on. Have your child sit on the potty seat while you read or offer a toy. Also, tune in to cues. Be aware of how your child behaves when he has to pee or poop. Look for a red face and listen for grunting sounds. Take notice of the time when he pees and poops during the day. Then establish a routine in which your child sits on the potty during those times, especially after meals or after drinking a lot of fluid. This helps set your child up for success.

And use plenty of praise, praise, and more praise. Is your child motivated by verbal encouragement? Stickers on a chart? Small toys or extra bedtime stories? Check in with what feels right for you and use it to reward positive potty choices. Your good attitude will come in handy, especially when "accidents" happen.

3.3 What Not to Do

Sitting on the potty should be a want-to, not a have-to. If your child isn't into it, don't force it.
Just when you think your child has nailed it, accidents happen. It's OK to be frustrated, but don't punish or shame your child -- it won't get you closer to your goal. Take a deep breath and focus on what you and your child can do better next time. Also, don't compare your son or daughter with other children. Some parents like to brag about how easy potty training went in their family. So if your neighbor says her kids potty trained themselves, smile and remember that the only right way is the one that works for you.

And if you a working mum, you juggle all your professional and personal responsibilities and, somehow, you make it look simple. Life is busy, though, and you've

got a huge task to add to the to-do list: learning how to potty-train.

Helping your little one switch from diapers to the bathroom is a tough job — regardless of whether you're a stay-at-home or working parent. Because you fall into

the latter category, you have to plan the process more carefully, so you are present for the majority of the transition. As you prepare for life without diapers, here are some tips to keep in mind to make it simpler for you as you balance your professional schedule and potty-train schedule.

1. Choose the Right Time

Parenting books will probably suggest the perfect time to start potty-training, but no two children are the same. Some little ones start using the potty at as young as 24 months, but that's rare. In most cases, children begin between 24 and 36 months, and the entire process can take up to eight months to perfect after that.

Still, you should be more focused on starting the process when your child shows they are ready for it. For instance, some kids will start to show interest in their siblings' or classmates' potty behavior, which can help you ease them into using the toilet, too. Also, if your child sleeps through nap time without wetting their diaper, they could be prepared to potty-train. To that end, staying dryer for longer also shows a little one has what it takes to wear big-kid underwear. Finally, your child might alert you when they must go, hide when they have to pee or poop, or tug at a dirty diaper. Once you

start seeing these cues, you should start thinking about beginning the process. There's no need to start too soon and put too much on your plate when you're already busy.

2. Invest in the Tools

Now that you know it's time to potty-train, you have to invest in the supplies you need to make it possible. For one thing, you'll need to pick up some underwear for your son or daughter. On a weekend or after-work trip to the store, bring your child along to help pick out their designs — they'll find it even more exciting to switch to underwear if they like the character or colors. Having the proper clothing and underwear, along with other potty-training supplies like extra bed sheets, flushable wipes, and soap you can keep your child comfortable and ready for anything.

However, mistakes happen! If they do make a mess, teach them to not put anything other than toilet paper or flushable wipes in the toilet! By preventing the flushing of wipes and the use of too much paper, you will minimize the amount of plumbing-related issues you will experience. When clogs do occur, knowing how to effectively use a plunger and when to call in a plumber can also save you a lot of grief.

3. Work with Teachers or Nannies

You can kick off your potty-training extravaganza over the weekend but, by Monday, you'll have to go back to work. Rather than halting your progress and popping your child back into diapers, work with their nanny or preschool teacher so everyone's on the same page about the transition. Chances are, your childcare provider will be more than willing to stick to the routine you've started, as well as any rewards system you have in place. Think about it — it's beneficial for them not have to change diapers anymore, either. Make sure you pack plenty of dry clothes just in case, as accidents do happen. Then, once you pick up your child and go home, you can continue the training process yourself.

4. Reward Good Potty Habits

Experts have varying opinions on rewarding children for their successful use of the potty. Some say it's a great way to boost their accountability, while others think the feeling of being clean and dry is reward enough. It's up to you whether or not you'll incentivize the process with treats, stickers or a potty-training chart.

No matter what, it's vital that you verbalize how proud you are of your child as they use the potty. Even if their teachers take the reins during the day, shower them

with praise as soon as you pick them up and hear updates on the process. It can be frustrating if your child fusses about using the toilet or if they suffer from accidents, but you can't let them see or feel this from you. With a supportive parent helming the transition from diapers to potty, children are more likely to try. Start and Succeed

Once you've pinpointed the right time to start, invested in the right gear and enlisted the help of your child's teachers, you're ready to potty-train.

You'll be surprised how these simple steps can make it so much easier to get the job done, even while you're working. Cheer your child to the finish line both of you will be freer and happier sans diapers, which is the best benefit of all.

3.4 How to Potty Train a Child with Special Needs as a mum

If you have a child with special needs, then you know that you may not be able to rely on the "typical" signs of potty training readiness. Kristen Raney from Shifting Roots shares her experience with potty training her son. Potty Training a Child on the Autism Spectrum First of all, don't read those stories about moms who potty train their children in three days!!! This will not work for our

children and will cause you so much stress!! Remember through this process that you are a good mom doing the best you can for your child.

Most of the moms of autistic children I know were not able to potty train their children before four, many of them five, and some of them never. It just depends where your child falls on the Autism Spectrum and what their particular sensory issues are. For context, our son would be considered to have Aspergers, but it's no longer a diagnosis and is now part of the Autism Spectrum. His body was ready to potty train around 2 1/2, but he had very intense fears about using the toilet. No bribe, game, song, or sticker chart in the world could get him to use it. He also was terrified to pee or poo in pre-K, daycare, or anywhere in public. We started by getting him trained to pee on the potty, and he hit that milestone by 3 1/2. I don't remember how, because it was so stressful that I've erased that time from my mind. I think it involved making him pee in his diaper in the bathroom, and slowly transferring that idea to the potty. Once he got that, he had to ask for a diaper if he wanted to poo, and go in his diaper in the bathroom. To get him trained all the way, it took a 90 minute battle of wills where I told him he could poop on the potty or on

the bathroom floor, it was entirely his choice. It was terrible. He chose the potty, glared at me like I was killing him. We bought him a Thomas train for the next three times he went on the potty, and a fourth one for keeping it up for a week. Yes, this sounds completely excessive and terrible, but he was 4 1/4 and we were at our wits end. I hope your journey is much less stressful than ours, but know that you're not alone! Don't take any flack from someone with a neurotypical kid who gives you grief about not having your child trained by now. You've got this mama!

3.5 How to Potty Train a "Late" Bloomer

Here's the thing. Out of all of my mom friends, not one of our kiddos potty trained at the same age/time. In my grandparent's era, children were toilet trained early (12-18 months). This had a lot to do with the needs of the adult, however, not necessarily the readiness of the child. Most American families are now waiting until their child is at least twenty-four months or beyond to introduce potty training. Keep in mind, that times are always changing!

An article by Healthy Children.org entitled "The Right Age to Potty Train", states that there is no exact right

age potty train! Research over the past several decades indicates that there is no perfect age. Parents really need to look at the physical, mental, and emotional readiness of their child and go from there. These indicators could happen at vastly different ages.

Sumer Schmitt over at Giggles, Grace, and Naptime shares her experiences with potty training on "older toddler". Her son was nearly three and a half when he was fully potty trained. She shares her story of persevering through potty training and advises:

We, as moms, have heard it a million times. Don't compare. Don't compare your child to little Suzy down the street who was potty trained at 18 months. Or the story you read online about the 6 month old baby who is already doing elimination communication. Easier said than done, right? When you're in the thick of it though, it's hard not to get stuck in the comparison game.

Trust me, I get it. But, your child will potty train in his/her own time. Chances are, by the time your child reaches kindergarten, no one is even going to be talking about this milestone anymore. Just like they no longer talk about when your child first rolled over, sat up, crawled, or started walking. Those milestones are in the past and most children will all eventually catch up to one

another. Studies actually show that sometimes potty training later is better because your child will have a better developed vocabulary. Potty training may be easier and happen faster the later the age!

3.6 How to potty train your kid as a dad

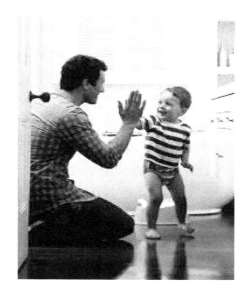

As a father, either single father or not our child is more likely to understand potty use if he's no longer wearing a nappy. Training pants are absorbent underwear worn during toilet training. They're less absorbent than nappies but are useful for holding in bigger messes like accidental poos. Once your child is wearing training pants, dress her in clothes that are easy to take off quickly. Pull-ups are very popular and are marketed as helpful for toilet training. It isn't clear that they actually help. But you can try them to help your child get used to

wearing underwear. Generally, cloth training pants are less absorbent than pull-ups and can feel a little less like a nappy. Pull-ups might be handier when you're going out. Wearing training pants is a big move for your child. If you celebrate it, the transition will be easier. Talk about how grown-up he is and how proud of him you are. I've heard all the tricks stickers, bribing with toys, special underpants. But you have to pick something that's consistent with your parenting style. I didn't use rewards elsewhere, so I didn't want to start here. What did work: Lots of undivided attention, positive reinforcement, love, affection and pride when my kids were successful. Making a big deal about small steps of progress is key. I didn't use any special stuff—no kiddie toilets, potty rings, or even pull-ups—because the local YMCA where my daughters attended didn't believe in them. We even had to sign a contract stating that we'd follow their potty training policy at home. I was instructed to just put the kids (they were around 2 1/2) on our regular toilet throughout the day when I thought they had to go. After a week and lots of "Yeah! You did number two!" and "Good for you! You made a wee-wee!" they were done, with barely any accidents. All told, I think they were just developmentally ready. "The key is consistency," says James Singer, father of two, and a member of the Huggies Pull-Ups Potty Training Partners. "Whatever you do at home with your potty training plan, you also need to do elsewhere. For instance, if your child prefers to read a book while on the potty, talk to your daycare provider about sending in a favorite book. Keep in mind that daycare centers may be too busy to customize potty training to each child. In that case, ask them how they think they can help foster the success you have had at home and compromise. Then bring home something that works at daycare. If your child loves the soap they use at school, get some for home. Boost the fun factor of using the potty with a Pee-Kaboo Reusable Potty Training Sticker. Slap a blank sticker onto the base of a portable potty, have your toddler pee in the potty, and then let him watch as an image of a train, flower, fire truck, or butterfly appears! After you empty, clean, and dry the potty, the image disappears, ready to be used again and again for up to six weeks. Too good to be true? We tested it on a formerly reluctant potty trainer, 2-year-old Gwenyth Mencel, who now shouts "Butterfly, butterfly!" when it's time to hit the potty. Are you counting down the days to the toilet transition? Or maybe you've already dabbled in a few less-than-successful attempts? Either way, we heard one thing again and again: Your kid has to be good and ready. And don't worry, he will be someday. "No child is going to graduate high school in diapers," says Carol Stevenson, a mom of three from Stevenson Ranch, California, who trained each one at a different age. "But it's so easy to get hung up and worried that your child's a certain age and not there yet, which adds so much pressure and turns it into a battle." Once you're convinced your kid's ready to ditch the diapers (watch for signs like showing an interest in the bathroom, telling you when she has to go, or wanting to be changed promptly after pooping), try any of these tricks to make it easier.

3.7 An explanation from an experience Dad

My wife, MJ, and I ran into the usual parent challenges when trying to potty-train our son. At first Will, then 2, was confused, then afraid, and next defiant. At 2 1/2 he still loved that diaper, and the mere sight of a toilet sent him into a tantrum. The most frustrating part was that I knew he was ready. He would stay dry the entire night, wake up, and pee into his diaper while standing right in front of us, grinning. It was a not-so-subtle reminder

that if Will was going to learn, it would be on his own terms. MJ and I spent countless hours trying to make the bathroom more appealing. We brought Will's stuffed animals in there, let him flip through his books while sitting on the potty (good training for when he's older, like Dad), and even threw Cheerios in the bowl to give him a target. Nothing worked.

At last we got Will to stand on the stool, lift up the seat, pull his pants down, and loom over the toilet. But he still wouldn't go. "Dad, it's not working," he'd say in the cutest way imaginable.

At first I urged him to keep trying. No go. So I turned on the faucet, thinking the sound of running water would make him feel like peeing. But I forgot that he doesn't like noise, so this move merely upset him. Finally I had a eureka moment. "Hey, Bud, how 'about if Dad pees with you, and we race?" I said. This clearly sparked Will's competitive spirit, because he brightened up and agreed to the challenge. I shifted his stool to the right so I could squeeze in next to him, and we prepared for our duel. I told him we'd fire on the count of three. But my little cheater jumped the gun. I didn't even get to "two" before he let loose a stream into the toilet. Victory. Will giggled and grinned with pride, and I silently awarded

myself first place in the "Best Dad in the Universe" contest for solving the potty-training riddle. I smiled broadly at father and son sharing a moment, hitting a milestone (er, Cheerio), and having some genuine fun.

A little too much fun, as it turns out. Will became so excited and began laughing so hard that he started falling in mid-spritz. I was still peeing as well, so I did my best to keep him balanced, all the while making sure we hit the porcelain bull's-eye. Will's left foot slipped off the stool. I was able to catch him somewhat with my hip and right hand, but not before he instinctively turned toward me. Yup, that's right he sprayed me. A good father would've taken the punishment. But I'm squeamish, so I jerked my body away from his shower. That caused my own pee to hit the wall and ricochet onto my poor son's back.

We both fell to the floor, shocked and disgusted. We were silent for a moment, until Will spoke.

"Dada?" he said quizzically. "Yes, Bud?" "You peed on me." "To be fair, you peed on me first."

The two of us started cracking up belly laughs, guffaws, cackling, you name it - to such a degree that I would have peed myself right there if I hadn't just soaked my toddler. The racket attracted the attention of MJ, who came rushing over. When she turned the corner she stared at us: our soaked clothes, the yellow droplets slowly making their way down the wall.

I launched into an explanation. "Honey, you see, there was a pee race ..." "I don't care," she interrupted, turning on her heels and walking away. "Just clean it up."

I did, and that day turned out to be a breakthrough. Will began using the toilet regularly (he asked me many times to race him again, but I never accepted) and was fully trained less than two months later. The bad news? He can't resist the urge to tell anyone and everyone about the time Dad peed on him.

3.8 How to Potty train a kid as a grandpa

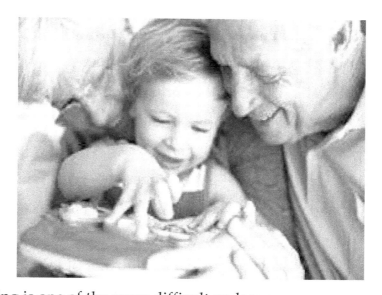

Potty training is one of the more difficult endeavors we face as old parents. Every child is different and has their own unique challenges. Unfortunately, it's a messy, stinky destination that you'll quickly want to conquer, but will seemingly get stuck in the mud (no pun intended). So why do some grand parents struggle so much with potty training? The answer may be in the diversity, or lack there of our teachings. The way I see it, the more activities you do to promote potty usage, the better your child's chance of success. You have to stack the deck in your favor. Some parents only do one or two things like buy pull-ups and attempt to put their child on the potty until they get frustrated from it not working. There is a better way. In fact, several different ways which should all be used in conjunction to make potty time a little less night marish and actually more successful!

Children are typically ready to potty train around the ages of 2 or 3 but maybe earlier if there are older siblings to learn from. Look for the signs. Look out for signs that your child is ready. These include pulling their diaper on and off, going a while or whole nap with a dry diaper, telling you they're going, showing curiosity about the potty and what goes in it, and going number 2 the same time each day. When starting, dedicate 1-2 weeks to potty training. This includes pausing play-dates, car rides, outdoor activities, and basically anything that brings your child out of the house. Once you start, there's no turning back. Make sure you're in it for the long haul...all or nothing. Avoid pull-ups during the day as they give children a crutch to go, just like a diaper. Instead, let them be naked and rush them to the potty if they start to go while saying, "Make sure you go pee pee in the potty."

Put them on the potty every 15 to 30 minutes. A lot of kids also have a set time of day when they do their "number 2" business. Make sure to put your child on the potty for several minutes during this time of day and encourage them to go number 2.

Make it enticing and convenient for them to go by providing a smaller, fun themed potty that's not so intimidating to a toddler. My son had a fire truck potty that he loved and we kept it in the room he would play in. Teach the process of going potty and washing hands with books! There are a ton of great books that you can read to your toddler while sitting on the potty.

Make a cool potty earning chart with fun stickers and rewards. My son received a sticker every time he went potty and after eight stickers he received a little cheap

toy like a matchbox car. You can also reward with a few mini M&Ms when they're successful. Charts are a great way to be consistent. Nighttime potty training usually comes later. We put nighttime pull-ups on our toddler for a good six months after he was day time potty trained. It wasn't until he started going the entire night without incident did we stop using them. Try your best to stay calm, use positive reinforcement, and not get angry or frustrated when they have an accident. You don't want your child to be anxious or stressed with potty time. Don't make them feel bad for having an accident. They might not tell you when it happens the next time. As stated earlier, potty training is one of the most difficult parts of being a parent. Consistency is your friend in this situation. Don't give up. Even with hard work, regression is possible and normal. Keep working at it until your little one is a potty pro.

Chapter 4 How to potty train your kid in 3 days

The "Signs of Readiness"

I've heard people say that the child needs to show "signs of readiness" before you can potty train them for 3 days.

This is true. What most people don't understand is, "What exactly is a sign of readiness"? People often say that a sign of readiness is when the child starts showing interest in the toilet more than usual. In my opinion, this is an enormous misconception.

Children are curious creatures. As soon as they can crawl, they're out exploring their world. They inevitably find the toilet bowl and start playing in   the   water.

This is not "the sign" to look for (though it is if you want to prevent them from getting sick, hurt or causing other mayhem). A necessary sign of potty training readiness is the ability for the child to frequently communicate his or her wants. I'm not talking about speech. I'm talking about gestures, behaviors, sounds, signing. If you can understand that a child wants something, and the child can direct you to the item, that is good enough. Believe me, when a child is pulling your leg into the kitchen or bedroom, they know what they want, and they are

effectively communicating with you! There is greater significance in this sign than you might think. What this behavior or attribute also means is that many children with Apraxia or speech, autism and other developmental problems can be potty trained using this method. Ultimately, the child learns that using the toilet is a good thing, something to be rewarded, and they will find a way to communicate their need to you. They like being rewarded. A parent explained: My fifth child was diagnosed with Childhood Apraxia of Speech and was potty trained at 22 months old in under 3 days using 3 Day potty training method this is not an easy task. At the time his vocabulary consisted mainly of sounds - not actual words. If a child with apraxia can use potty at 22 month why did you think your own kid cant do that. Secondly, your child must be able to go to bed without a bottle or cup, preferably two to three hours before bedtime.

4.1 There are a couple reasons why I say this.

1)I care about your child's dental health 2)It makes for easy potty training What happens to you when you have a lot to drink just

before going to bed? Late night visits to the bathroom! The same goes for your child. If you give them lots of fluid before bed, there's little chance they will wake up dry.

4.2 A few common questions I get from moms about this sign of readiness:

1)Our dinner is only an hour before bed, do I not give my child anything to drink? It is just fine for you to give your child something to drink with dinner. Just be sure that he's not getting tons just before he goes down for the night.

2)My child really enjoys his cup of milk before bed as it is part of our night time routine. Do I really need to stop this? No, you can continue as you have milk with your night time routine but try to decrease the amount. To do this maybe you can get him a smaller cup and then only fill it half way full. Also be sure to follow the night time routine outlined in this eBook.

3)My child wakes often during the night needing a drink, I don't want to tell him no because it's really dry where we live. You can go ahead and let your child have his "sips" of water during the night if he really needs this but there is no need for full cups of water. Being that

your child does wake for drinks, he shouldn't have a problem also getting up to go to the bathroom.

Third, in order for this method to work for children under the age of 22 months of age, your child must be waking up dry. Check for dryness within half an hour of them waking up. Don't wait until they've been up for an hour or so. By then, they will have peed and you won't get an accurate indication of readiness. If your child is over the age of 22 months old he should be waking up dry but don't worry too much if he does not. Just be sure to follow the night time method outlined in the eBook to help him with waking up dry.

4.3 A few common questions I get from moms about this sign of readiness:

1)My child is 3 years old and still wakes up with a full

diaper. Can I still potty training my child? Yes! As stated above, if your child or grandchild is over the age of 22 months and they still wake up wet, it's ok. Just be sure to follow the night time steps outlined in the eBook.

2)My first child is 5 years old and still wets the bed, I don't think my 2 year old will be able to be potty trained for nights. Can I just potty train for the days and use a pull-up or diaper for nights? Why would you want to?

There is no need. You can easily potty train your child (even your older child) to wake up dry if you follow the method outlined in the eBook. It works!

3) My child is 18 months old and shows most the signs of readiness but doesn't wake up dry; can I still start potty training? Yes, just be sure to

follow the steps outlined in the eBook for night time. I do recommend waiting until your child is 22 months of age because it can take longer than three days when they are younger than 22 months, but the choice is yours. It is my experience that children 22 months of age are at the ideal age to be potty trained. It is entirely possible that a 15 month old shows these signs. For me, if my 15 month old showed these signs, I would still wait until 22 months.

4.4 The First day Journey to the 3 days potty training

Day 1 is the day that we decide to start potty training. First of all, as mentioned earlier, make sure that not only you, but also your child and anyone else who's involved, gets a good night's rest. This is extremely important. It's very difficult to accomplish something when you are not only tired but the child is tired and everyone is cranky.

It is on this day that you get rid of the diapers and the child starts wearing big boy and big girl underwear fulltime... There are no more diapers in this process... Now, some of you are saying, "Well, maybe we'll go ahead and use pull-ups or padded underwear." What I like to say is, "A diaper is a diaper no matter what you call it or what you disguise it as." And subconsciously, if you put the diaper on the child, it gives them the wrong message. Also, seeing as that we've already explained how difficult this process is for the parents or the potty trainer as it is for the child, not having the diaper makes the parent or the potty trainer more vigilant. You will pay more attention if you know that the child does not have a diaper on.

For example, if you know the child has a diaper and you are out and about somewhere in a store or going out shopping you might say to yourself, "Well, we don't have to find a bathroom right now. We're kind of in a rush.

You've got a diaper on." But note that the one time you tell that child that it's okay to go potty in that diaper; you have opened Pandora's Box. You've just told them, "its okay". And they will continue to do that and you will hit a lot of regressions. So, we start with allowing them to pick their big boy or girl underwear and put it on.

(This is something you might have done during the pre-potty training process).

Then, you're going to sit down with your child and explain the process to them again. You can say, "Here's what we are doing; here is what Mommy expects; and here is what's going to happen." Then, you'll want to let them pick the spot for their potty chair.

You'll ask them, "Where do you want your potty chair?" We want to give them some control as well. If you have 2 bathrooms in the house, let them pick their favorite bathroom if they're going to be using the bathroom instead of the potty chair.

Then, you're going to take them to the bathroom. They are going to sit on the toilet and you are going to say, "Okay, Mommy wants you to use the bathroom." By this point, they should have seen you use the bathroom, so you can also say, "We want you to use the bathroom just like Mommy uses the bathroom." Don't be disappointed if nothing comes out. The act that getting them to sit there is a reward or it's an accomplishment all on its own. Once they get off the toilet, you're going to set a timer for 20 minutes.

Every 20 minutes for the first 3 days or for the first few days until they're trained, you are going to have them

go and sit in the bathroom. When the timer goes off (and this is very important) it almost has to become a celebration in the house. Everybody can clap or say, "It's potty time. It's potty time. Let's go potty." And everyone can run to the bathroom.

Even with our older kids when we were potty training our youngest, would join into the celebration and run to the bathroom. And it was as if it was Cinco de Mayo or some big festivity in the house. That is very important because we're trying to make this a fun experience for the child.

Every time they go to the bathroom at those 20 minute intervals, you want to make sure they sit on the toilet for 3 to 5 minutes. This is not about them sitting on the toilet for hours; it's sitting on the toilet for 3 to 5 minutes. If they go right away and they pee or they do number 2, then they can get up right away.

Now, if they don't do either one then you want to make sure you wait the full 5 minutes with them sitting on the toilet. Note: At this point, we are not so much concerned about number 2. We want you and them to master number 1 first and then we'll move on. Now, even if they don't go, that is okay because the fact that you're getting them to sit down on the toilet is, again, an

accomplishment all in its own. But something that you want to see happen every single time they sit down on the toilet is for them to push. Even if they don't go number 2 or they don't do number 1, you want to make sure they push. So, you'll want to say, "Mommy wants to see you push. Now push." And some parents have told us, "Well, I can't tell when they're pushing." What you want to do is look at their stomach.

You can tell by the stomach muscle flexing whether they are pushing or not. You see, with a child, it is impossible for them to hold and push at the same time. So, you're almost tricking them into using the potty by asking them to push. So, no matter what—no matter where you go, no matter what time it is—the minute they sit on the toilet you want to make sure that they push and they push every single time. Even if nothing comes out, as long as they push, that is a good thing because we want to get them used to using those muscles and pushing and moving whatever is inside of their system out. If you find they do not understand what pushing is, what you can do is just tickle their stomachs and the tickling sensation will cause them to contract their stomach muscles, which is a natural way to push.

The other thing that you want to start doing is giving

them more fluids. Many people think that potty training is about not wetting themselves. That is not what potty training is about. Potty training is about recognizing when you have to go and knowing where to do it. So, one of the things that you're going to do to help them recognize that is giving them more fluids. However, you do not want to give them more juice because sometimes the sugar and starches that are in the juice can cause constipation and other problems. Instead, you want to give them liquids like water and things that are going make them want to go potty. In addition to helping them potty, water also helps in the number 2 process as well, which we'll talk about later.

Now, sometimes what happens is that the child will sit for 5 minutes, they won't go, they'll get up and then they might wet themselves within a minute or two. So, here's what you do in that situation: shorten the amount of time that they sit on the toilet. Instead of sitting on the toilet for 5 minutes, let them sit on the toilet for 1 or 2 minutes, but you increase the frequency of how many times they go to the bathroom. So, instead of every 20 minutes, now it's every 15 minutes for 1 to 2 minutes. Another thing you'll want to do is ask them from the minute they get off the toilet and at least 3 or 4 times during that 20 minute timeframe, "Do you have to go potty? "Most of the time, they're going to tell you, "No," and that's okay.

You just want to get them used to hearing the words, "Do you have to go potty?" Then, when the 20 minutes are up and it's time to go potty, now the question is not, "Do you have to go potty?" Now, it's, "Time to potty."

One is asking and one is telling. Hopefully you see and understand the difference between the two statements. It's very, very important especially for psychologically getting the child to want to go and use the toilet.

4.5 Constipation

Alright, let's start with holding. Some children will actually hold number 2. Sometimes they will hold number 2 for a day or two days. When it finally becomes too painful they will let it all out into the diaper. First of all if you find your child is holding it that long and all the other methods are not working, and then put a diaper on to let them go. Holding bowel that long is not good for them. This is one of the rare times we recommend putting on a diaper. The thing to realize is...if they are holding it that long, then theoretically just by the nature of what potty training is, that says your child is potty

trained and know what to do. For whatever reason they are afraid of the potty. It's not an issue of potty training. It's an issue of being afraid or maybe going potty is too painful for them. If you find that their stool is hard, then it will lead to painful bowel movement. If they associate all bowels as painful then they would rather hold the stool then to let it go. So the things that you can do are give them foods that will cause them to go to the bathroom. Give them more liquids (preferably water, not soda or juice), more liquids in their system the easier for them to go number You want to also do other things. When they're sitting on the toilet try to take their mind off the potty. Some ways to do that would be to rub their stomach or their feet. In the scientific world this is called neuro-linguistic programming. Basically you are trying to get their mind off of something that they're afraid of. So by doing something that feels good to them, you are associating the toilet with something that feels good. Now they're not afraid of that anymore. You want to tickle them. When you tickle them, it forces them to push. You've heard me use the word push over and over so it's something that I'm going to stress. Make sure they push. As long as they push you are doing good. They cannot hold and push at the same time. I cannot stress enough how important pushing is. If you feel they don't know what pushing is, then tickle their stomach and that will help them understand what pushing is. The other thing that you want to look at when it comes number 2 is constipation. There are a lot of things that cause constipation. Some causes of constipation are medical, while other causes are more mental. If you find your child is constipated, you want to do what I call the "bicycle trick". Don't ask how we had figured this out, but this works 100% of the times. What you do is you lay your child on their back. You should kneel in front of your child at the base of their feet.

Their feet should be almost touching your lap. Grab the base of their feet. Then rotate their legs as if they're riding a bicycle. Do this for about 10 minutes. Within 25 -30 minutes of doing this, the child will use the bathroom. We've told many parents to do this. Every parent I've told to try this, we've gotten a 100% success rate, whereas the child will end up using the bathroom within 30 minutes of doing the "bicycle trick". So that is the constipation, and if you find the constipation lasting 4 or 5 days you may want to seek some form of medical attention for the child. That is not normal for them to be

able to hold it for that many days.

4.6 The second day journey of the 3 days

Alright, so you've graduated from number 1. Your child is doing very well using number 1. Now, it's time for them to start using number 2. There is not much difference between training them from number 1 to number 2. As a matter of fact, I would go so far to tell you that number 1 is a lot harder than number 2, and the reason being that when they go number 1, they have to actually take action to hold it inside. In other words, for them not to wet themselves, they have to actually squeeze the sphincter muscle and hold the fluids inside. Whereas with number 2, they don't have to do anything to hold it. They actually have to push it out so it is an action that is a lot less difficult than holding the number 1 is. This is behaviour. They have to actually take a step. They have to be proactive to go number 2 so they have a whole lot more control in the number 2 process than they do in number 1. Now, again, one of the things that we want to make sure we do when they're sitting on the toilet is pushing. And, hopefully you understand how important the pushing strategy is. No matter how far along in the potty training process whether they are two years old or whether they are four

and a half—pushing is extremely important because that is how they are training themselves to go. This is especially true when it comes to number 2. Now, some kids will want to go in number 2 in their diaper or a pull up. They will actually go and ask their parent for a pull up or a diaper to go number 2. Now, if this is the case for you, what you want to realize is the pull up then becomes a security blanket for the child.

In this case, what you might say is something to the effect of, "Okay, if you go number 2, then we'll put the pull up on." What that says is, "If you go number 2 first then we'll get the pull up." Now, something else I've had parents do is actually go get the pull up, let them put the pull up on only around their ankles. That way, they have their security blanket on, and they can feel it, and they can see it, yet they're sitting on the toilet. This allows them to use the bathroom and feel comfortable.

The other thing you want is to make sure that you give them is more fluids as I explained earlier. And you will also want to make sure to track their schedule. A lot of kids will go to the bathroom for number 2 at the same time or around the same time every day. With my youngest son, it was like clockwork. Within 30 minutes of him eating anything, he would go to use the potty and

do number 2. So, we always knew after he ate that he was going to use the bathroom. Using a potty training journal is helpful. If you don't have a potty journal and a potty chair or a potty chart, you can get yourself a potty training chart and journal to track when they go to the bathroom. Let's say you find that they go after dinner, which is around the time frame of 7:00 in the evening. Well, what happens is you're still using the same consistency as using number 1 which is every 20 minutes except now you are watching for 7 o'clock to come around because you know that they're going to be using the bathroom within a half hour. At this point, what you want to do is time the bathroom use. You want to get them on the toilet but you also want to make sure that they stay on the toilet long enough to use the bathroom or use the bathroom to do number 2. their underwear again. It's going to help them make sure they use the bathroom the next time they go.

4.7 When they finally get it right

Alright, now you're taking them to the bathroom every 20 minutes and you go 3 days and you are not getting any accidents. Don't make the mistake that most parents make as I mentioned very early on. This is the

stage when many parents decide that, "My child is potty trained and there was nothing left for me to do." This is the point in time where you want to be more consistent, more consistent, and more consistent.

This is when you want to make sure that you are still taking them to the bathroom every 20 minutes or you might change the interval from 20 minutes to 30 minutes. You might even feel comfortable waiting even longer than that - maybe 45 minutes. But don't let 45 minutes to an hour go by that you are not taking your child to the bathroom. Let me give you an example why this is. Your body has to get what's called "muscle memory." Remember at this point the child is only in stage 3 of potty training.

That's where they know what they're doing. They know what's wrong but they're thinking about it. It's not subconscious yet. At this point in time, the child is still thinking, "Should I go; should I not go? Where should I go? What should I do?" Think about it this way: Michael Jordan is one of the best basketball players that have ever played the game, yet even when he was scoring 30, 40, 50 points a game, he was still shooting and practicing for hours a day, taking 500 to 600 foul shots every single day. Even though he was the best there

was, he was still practicing harder than anybody else. That is the difference between regular athletes and professionals. The professionals, they practice harder than anybody else because when they get into a situation, they do not have to think about it, the body automatically reacts. So, that's why when your child is finally starting to get it, you have to then make sure you maintain the consistency.

Chapter 5 Getting them to tell you

How do you get them to start telling you? Basically the question is how do we get your child from Stage 3 to Stage 4? And Stage 4 is where they can go to the bathroom themselves. They recognize on their own, they don't need you to take them to the bathroom every 20 minutes. Basically, its complete autonomy and freedom for the child and complete autonomy and freedom for you... So, the question is, "How do we get to that stage?" With consistency. You have to be consistent.

Once they start to show you they are ready, you have to make sure that you are continually being consistent. The other thing you can do is you can play the game that I call the "let's race to the potty game." All you do is sit at the table with your child and you say, "Okay, let's see who can get to the potty first and whoever wins gets a prize." So, basically it's a race between you and the child, and, of course, you're going to let the child win (but they don't know that).

Then, you pick a good reward of something that they're going to enjoy or really like. To start the race they have to say the words, "Mommy, I have to go potty." That's the cue. It's like saying "1, 2, 3, set go." But instead of saying "1, 2, 3, set go," they say, "Mommy I have to go potty". Once they say that, the race begins, so the both of you run to the bathroom and the first one that gets to the bathroom wins the game. What this does is gets the child used to saying, "I have to go potty," and then the next steps are them going to the bathroom. You want to practice this probably two or three times a day once you find that they are starting to be more consistent with no accidents. You don't want to start this game while they're in the potty training process because they've got enough to worry about. So, you want to start this only after you've seen that they have finally gotten it and they're starting to do pretty well on their own.

5.1 How to Use Positive Practice for Accidents

Another useful technique is positive practice for accidents. Dr. Schaefer describes this as what you should do when your child has an accident and wets or soils himself. This technique involves firmly telling your child what he has done, taking him to the potty where he can clean and change himself (although you will likely need to help) and then having him practice using the potty. Dr. Schaefer recommends going through the usual steps of using the potty at least five times, starting

when "the child walks to the toilet, lowers his pants, briefly sits on the toilet (3 to 5 seconds), stands up, raises his pants, washes his hands, and then returns to the place where the accident occurred."

Although you are trying to teach him the consequences of having an accident, this should not take the form of punishment.

5.2 Children Tantrums

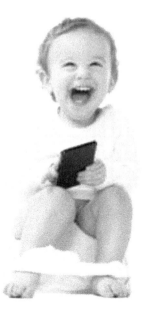

Tantrums are going to happen. A tantrum is frustration. That's the child not being able to verbally explain or talk about their emotion. So, the only way they know how to do that is through screaming and pitching a fit. Here's how you handle a tantrum... What you don't want to do is make potty training a battle. It's not a battle between

you and the child, but the child is trying to battle you. The child is trying to be in charge, and you're trying to be in charge at the same time. So, sometimes the way that you handle that is to totally ignore the tantrum. If your child is throwing a tantrum, you can walk away and say, "Mommy is not listening to you. Mommy will talk to you when you are calmed down," or "Mommy is not listening to you when your voice is louder than Mommy's." So you can turn around and use reverse psychology by turning the tables on your child. Once they have calmed down, you will want to say in a very strong and direct voice, "Mommy did not appreciate that," or "Grandma did not appreciate that," or "Daddy did not appreciate that behavior.

We expect better things. Let's go and try again." So, now you go right back to the basics and you take the child back to the bathroom and say, "We are going to use the bathroom and here's what we expect." If they throw a tantrum again, you walk away.Mind you, while that tantrum is going on, do not give them any rewards. Do not allow them to play with their toys. They are not allowed to do any of that fun stuff that they normally would want to do because you want to associate that tantrum with a bad behavior that results in loosing

something. So, the most important thing I can tell you is to ignore the tantrum, don't pay attention to it because as the laws of physics say, "For every action, there's an equal and opposite reaction." If you react to that tantrum, they are going to react to you. Once you react, they react. You react again, they react and it's going to escalate even more. So, the easiest way to squash it is not to put in the energy toward that tantrum. Once the child feels and sees that they're not getting energy out of you, then they realize that they're getting nothing by throwing this tantrum and there's nothing to be gained from it.

5.3 Regression in potty Training

What is a regression? A regression is a child that was potty trained, they were doing well, or they were starting to do well and for whatever reasons, they have done an about-face. Now, they are wetting themselves or they are soiling their diapers with poop. The question is "What really is the regression? What are the cause and the root of that regression?" These are the issues that need to be dealt with. Usually a regression is not so much an issue with potty training, but it's an emotional issue. The child will regress as a way to get attention or as a way of expression. So, most parents deal with regression by dealing with potty training, but the reality is the best way to deal with a regression is to try to find the underlying root cause. It could be one of many things causing the regression. A new baby being born, you've moved, a friend has moved, a family member might have passed away... Something has happened in that child's life and they don't know how to express it except through regression.

Something that a lot of parents have asked is, "When it comes to potty training, we've got a new baby on the way, should I wait to have the baby or will they regress if I potty train them and then we have the baby?" The best thing to do is to potty train them now. It is a lot easier to retrain a child that has been trained and has gone through a regression than it is to try to train a child that has never been trained. In addition to that as a parent, if you are having a new baby coming, you do not want to have a new baby and potty training duties at the same time. That's very, very, difficult. What I always tell parents is that they'll only need two to three days to get the child to Stage 3. Stage 4 is what will take you a couple of days from there. Some kids even get to Stage 4 in one day. But the key is, take the two or three days,

get your child to Stage 3, then through consistency, work toward getting them to Stage 4. When the new baby comes, or whatever that activity is — whether it's a vacation or a move — if they do regress, they've already been trained. Getting them back and reversing the regression is going to be a lot easier than if you had never started at all. So what you want to do when your child does regress is you go back to the basics. This includes them being on the toilet every 20 minutes for 3-5 minutes. They will continue to do that until they stop the regressive behavior. The only time our youngest had a regression, I went on a business trip with Greg. Lorenzo had been fully potty trained for about three months both day and night. Then I went on that business trip with my husband, and Lorenzo went to stay at Grandma's. We only were gone Thursday, Friday, and Saturday and came back on Sunday. When we returned, it was as if this child had never seen a potty chair or had been potty trained in his life. Now I have no idea what happened in those four days. Maybe Grandma had let him do whatever he wanted, I do not know. Or maybe he just said, "You know what? You guys left me, and I'm going to fix you guys." Basically, we took him back to the basics, went back to every 20 minutes with him on the toilet. And within about a day, he was back to normal. But it was a little scary seeing that happen.

5.4 Addressing fear in the kids

What you want to do is separate the difference between a fear of the toilet and potty training. Many of the parents that we have worked with have lumped the two into one category by saying that the fear of the toilet is a potty training problem. The reality is that a fear of the toilet has nothing to do with potty training, and, in most cases, it is a fear of the toilet as we noted earlier. So what you have to do is address that fear by sitting and asking your child. Don't be afraid to do this. Just ask them what they are afraid of. Sometimes it might not be the potty training, but something else. One of the things that you can do to help your child if there is a fear of the toilet is get yourself a potty chair or potty seat insert. An insert is actually put into the toilet and the child can sit on that toilet instead of the adult seat, which is especially helpful if the child is a little bit smaller.

They are usually colorful and have giraffes on them and dinosaurs. There is also a handle so the child can hold on to the handle and balance themselves. This will help them feel safe and comfortable without the fear of falling into the toilet. Placing a step stool under their feet will also assist them in this area. But, if you find that they have a fear of the toilet, then a potty training chair will be the way to go instead of the insert.

Now the question is this, if there's a fear of the toilet, what is the cause of that fear? Sometimes it can be pain that the child has when they are going to the bathroom. This is especially true with number 2. So the question is, have they ever had diarrhea or have they ever had a diaper that was on too long which caused a skin irritation? They are now associating the toilet and potty with that pain.

It might possibly be constipation. As an adult, constipation can be very painful. So, think about the child. It also might not be actual constipation, but some kids naturally have hard stools and letting that go can be extremely painful for them. If that is the case, you want to make sure that you take a look when your child does use the bathroom more if they are in their diaper. Is their stool harder or is it soft? Was there any illness like the stomach virus or anything that caused them some pain? These are all the things that can cause the child to be not only fearful of the toilet, but can also cause a child to regress. So you want to be careful about this and ask yourself whether any of this has happened.

If you find the child has hard stool, one of the things that you can do is start giving the child more water, less sugar, and less starchy items, which will help them become hydrated. When the body becomes dehydrated, it will start to pull any fluids that it can get wherever it can get it. One of the places that it pulls the fluid from is going to be the stomach and the intestines. And once those fluids are pulled out, the result is hardened stool. Once that stool becomes hard it's going to be very difficult and very painful for that child to go to the bathroom. So having fluids in the system will help give him or her softer stool. Something else that you can do if there is a fear of the toilet is calling it by a different name. Instead of calling it "potty," you can give it another name that doesn't bear a negative connotation. Something simple might be, "Let's go push."

Another thing that will help you make the experience more enjoyable for the child is to place books by the toilet. You should also have some toys in the bathroom or let them bring some toys with them so that it's a comfortable environment and something that is more fun for them. Again, the key is making it a loving time and not a stressful time. If you can read to them or let

them look at picture books, it turns into more of an enjoyable process and a less stressful process.

5.5 Potty training Twins or multiple children

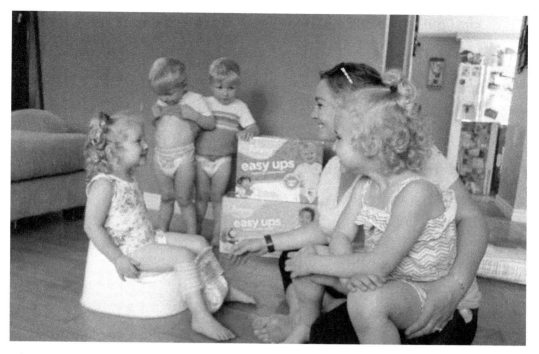

I have many parents with twins or multiples ask if this method can work for them. I also have parents with children at two different ages ask if the children can be potty trained simultaneously. The answer to both of these situations is "YES". You can potty train twins, multiples and two or more children at the same time. It's more demanding on you, and may take a few extra days, but it can be done.

If I, personally, had to choose between potty training multiples simultaneously or doing it one-at-a-time, I

would bite the bullet and do them all at the same time; "just be done with it." Having someone to help out is by far the best way. Be sure they read the guide. Discuss with them how you want situations handled. The two of you need to handle things identically. You can go it alone if you need to. Just be mentally prepared for some extra work. Also, the children must be right by your side at all times. If one child needs to use the restroom, ask the other child to come with. The underlying principle for potty training two or more children simultaneously is that you need to treat each child as an individual. Ideally, each child should have their own potty chair. They should each have their own underclothes and their own favorite treats and favorite drinks. Be sure to not use one's successes against the other child or children. Don't say things like, "See, Johnny can do it. Now you need to too." Just because one child might catch on right away doesn't mean that the other child / children will get it the first day or two. Keep in mind that they are individuals and that they may catch on at different times.

5.6 Help from daycare provider

If your child is in daycare be sure to discuss with your

daycare providers your plan a day or two before you start. Explain to them that when your child returns to daycare that they are not to put a pull-up or diaper on the child. They may come back to you and say that if the child has an accident, they will put a diaper on the child.

Gently remind them about the importance of being consistent, about how that would send mixed signals to the child, and could undo all the progress you've worked so hard to achieve, and that you greatly appreciate their support. Maybe even offer a pair of movie tickets. You or your spouse may need to take Friday or Monday off from work to give this method the best possible chance for success. Do not put your child in daycare during the three days. It's just too soon.

Day 4 is the earliest that I recommend returning your child to daycare.

Sometimes you may just have to play it by ear. At the end of day 3, if the whole toilet thing has not "clicked" with your child, you may need to take the next day off from work. The "clicking" or "getting it" needs to occur before the child returns to daycare. If your daycare provider is not on board with you then you might have a set back or two. I've never had my kids in daycare but many of the moms that I've helped potty train have kids in daycare. There are many wonderful daycare providers out there and they are willing to work with the parents but there are some that want nothing to do with helping the parents out. They want the child in a pull-up or diaper until they leave for school. If your daycare provider is one that isn't willing to support you during this training you might need to spend an extra day or two at home to make sure that there are no more accidents and that the child is confident in his new skill. You may need to be firm with your daycare provider with regards to your "no diaper" position.

If you are concerned about your daycare provider putting a pull-up or diaper back on your child, you might want to try Pods. Pods are little thin strips you place in your little ones underwear. These strips will absorb any accident your child has so he doesn't make a "mess" on the floor. Your child will feel the strips turn to a cold jell like substance and asked to go to the bathroom. The daycare provider can then just replace the strip. Pods can be the solution for those hard to work with daycare providers.

5.7 Travelling and Errands during potty Training

Alright, let's face the fact. You are a busy Mom or busy Dad or a busy Grandparent or a busy potty trainer. But you don't want to be stuck in the house during that potty training process. And yes —for a day or two you might be. But don't let potty training keep you from enjoying life and having fun and doing the things that you got to do. You may have shopping to do and errands to run. You might have a family to take care of. You've got things that you need to do. So here are some tips that will help you have a more successful potty training experience especially when you have things that you need to do.

First of all, you want to get yourself a spill-proof travel potty. If you don't have one, try to get one online travel and get yourself a spill-proof travel potty. Basically, it is a simple little potty chair which has a spill-proof lid. With that, you can keep it in the car so instead of having to be home to go to the bathroom every 20 minutes. You can be in the mall, you can be at the grocery store, you can be out shopping, and your child can still use the potty without the fear of having accidents. When you are

travelling or you're going to run errands, what you want to do is just like with the day care scenario, you want to use the bathroom before you leave. You will also want to plan your day and where you will be going so you'll be prepared about whether or not those places have bathrooms.

In other words, if you are going to place A and they have a bathroom and place B, does not have a bathroom, then you want to go to place B first right when you leave the house because your child has just gone. Once we would get to a location like a grocery store or a mall, especially if this is a grocery store or a mall that you've never been to, we would find the bathroom. So now, let's say we are out in the middle of shopping and Lorenzo had to go to the bathroom. It's wasn't a problem.

As soon as he said he had to go to the bathroom or we said, "Lorenzo, do you have to go to the bathroom?" and he said, "Yes," we knew where the bathrooms were. Most parents don't take that one step so what happens is the child says, "I have to go to the bathroom," the parents are in a state of panic to find the bathrooms. So, when we first got to the store, we would find the bathroom and then go to the bathroom. We would then get our most important stuff done first because we knew we just went to the bathroom and had more free time now than we might later. So, the smaller, less important things could wait. Back to the travel potty, these are really great because they will also help you out when you are going to take a long road trip. If you don't have one, you know that stopping frequently is going to be an issue. When Lorenzo was 2 years and 2 weeks, we had him fully potty trained and we took a trip to Florida. Back then, we were at Code Orange, and the government said it wasn't a good idea to fly. So, we decided to take a bus with three kids from Connecticut to Florida. It was a thirty-hour bus ride with a child that just finished potty training. To tell you it was a challenge is an understatement. Back then, there weren't spill-proof potty chairs so we didn't have one to bring, so we bought a huge 2 litre bottle. Every 20 minutes on the bus, we would hide in the corner or go into to the back and say, "Okay Lorenzo, pee into the bottle," and that's what he did. When he had to go number 2 luckily for us, was during a rest stop. But we didn't let the fact that he had the potty train keep us from doing what we had to do.

Chapter 6 Naptime and Nighttime Training

6.1 Naptime

Yes it's ok to put your child down for a nap during training. I personally have found that most kids will not have an accident if you have them go pee before the nap and then just as they wake up. Make sure you stay close though so you know when your child wakes.

6.2 Nighttime

Do not give your child anything to drink when they are getting ready for bed. In fact, it's best to stop the liquids 2 to 3 hours beforehand. Take them to the toilet at least twice before tucking them in to bed for the night. If nothing happens in the bathroom, maybe read a book together for a few minutes and try again. Remember what I said about "trying" don't keep them on the toilet. Having them clear their bladder is important. Once your child has released twice you can put them in bed. Do not use a diaper (you shouldn't have any).

If your child has a hard time waking up dry and they are older than 22 months, the following procedure may help Wake the child 1 hour after he or she has gone to sleep Take them to the toilet and return them to bed In the morning, wake the child 1 hour before they normally

arise Take them to the toilet This helps the child realize two things: 1)It is ok to get up to go pee 2)It is also expected If your child is in a crib, you can still follow these steps. You just need to keep an ear open for them. If you hear your child stirring, or whimpering, they may need to pee. You do not need to do the above steps if your child usually wakes up dry. Your child may wet the bed at night. Don't be alarmed or upset.

This is halfway to be expected – we're giving them lots of liquid. Don't make a big deal of it – don't reprimand or scold. Just change the sheets. Remind the child to tell you when he needs to go pee, and that they need to keep their underwear dry. Again, don't be negative; don't say "Bad, No," etc.

This will be the end of a busy and perhaps frustrating day. Do not worry. It will click; your child will "get it", if not tomorrow, then on the third day. Be sure to keep a positive and loving attitude with your child, even if you have to change sheets in the middle of the night.

A tip for parents with older children: To help your child to go to the bathroom before bed and to stay dry during the night you can try using a chart system with the

following on it:

6.3 Bedtime Routine:

go pee

put on night clothes

read a book

brush teeth

go pee again

keep bed dry all night

Let your child know that if he gets a star by each one he will get a prize in the morning.

Remind him that he's got to get up and go pee if he's got to go. A special tip, that works for even the hardest of cases. The following has been used even with long time bed-wetters to help them overcome bed wetting... Once your child goes to sleep, make a bed up on the floor without him knowing. Now throughout the night you will say to him "be sure to tell mommy when you have to go pee". Anytime during the night when you hear him start to move and stir around, say to him "Do you have to go pee? Make sure tell mommy when you have to go pee". What this does is allows you to see how often your child is stirring in his bed and will help him remember that he's suppose to pee in the potty not in

his bed.

6.4 Toddler discipline and proper upbringing

Have you ever found yourself in deep negotiations with your 2-year-old over whether she can wear her princess costume to preschool for the fifth day in a row? Have you taken the "walk of shame" out of the local supermarket after your toddler threw a temper tantrum on the floor? There may be comfort in knowing you're not alone, but that doesn't make navigating the early years of discipline any easier.

Toddlerhood is a particularly vexing time for parents because this is the age at which children start to become more independent and discover themselves as individuals. Yet they still have a limited ability to communicate and reason.

Child development specialist Claire Lerner, director of parenting resources for the nonprofit organization Zero to Three, says, "They understand that their actions matter -- they can make things happen. This leads them to want to make their imprint on the world and assert themselves in a way they didn't when they were a baby. The problem is they have very little self-control and they're not rational thinkers. It's a very challenging combination." What do you do when your adorable toddler engages in not-so-adorable behavior, like hitting the friend who snatches her toy, biting Mommy, or throwing her unwanted plate of peas across the room? Is it time for...timeout?

Timeout -- removing a child from the environment where misbehavior has occurred to a "neutral," unstimulating space -- can be effective for toddlers if it's used in the right way, says Jennifer Shu, MD, an Atlanta pediatrician, editor of Baby and Child Health and co-author of Food Fights: Winning the Nutritional

Challenges of Parenthood Armed With Insight, Humor, and a Bottle of Ketchup and Heading Home With Your Newborn: From Birth to Reality.

"Especially at this age, timeout shouldn't be punitive. It's a break in the action, a chance to nip what they're doing in the bud."

Timeouts shouldn't be imposed in anger, agrees Elizabeth Pantley, president of Better Beginnings, a family resource and education company in Seattle, and author of several parenting books, including The No-Cry Discipline Solution. "The purpose of timeout is not to punish your child but to give him a moment to get control and reenter the situation feeling better able to

cope." It also gives you the chance to take a breath and step away from the conflict for a moment so you don't lose your temper.

6.5 Timeouts is Not for Every Kid

Some experts insist that timeouts work for all, but Shu and Pantley disagree. "For some kids who just hate to be alone, it's a much bigger punishment than it's worth, especially with young toddlers," says Shu. "They get so upset because you're abandoning them that they don't remember why they're there, and it makes things worse." She suggests holding a child with these fears in a bear hug and helping her calm down.

You can also try warding off the kind of behavior that might warrant a timeout with "time-in." That means noticing when your children's behavior is starting to get out of hand and spending five or 10 minutes with them before they seriously misbehave. "It's like a preemptive strike," Shu says. "Once they've gotten some quality time with you, you can usually count on reasonably OK behavior for a little while."

6.6 Toddler Discipline Dos & Don'ts

Shu says a good stage to initiate timeouts is when your toddler is around age 2. Here are a few guidelines.

Do remove your child from the situation. Do tell him what the problem behavior was. Use simple words like "No hitting. Hitting hurts."Don'tberateyourchild. Do place her in a quiet spot -- the same place every time, if possible. For young toddlers, this may have to be a play yard or other enclosed space.

Don't keep him there long — the usual rule of thumb is one minute per year of age. Do sit down with your child after timeout is over and reassure her with a hug while you "debrief" by saying something like, "We're not going to hit anymore, right?" Don't belabor what the child did wrong. Instead, ask her to show you how she can play nicely.

6.7 Commandments Discipline for Toddler

Children aren't born with social skills it's human nature for them to start out with a survival-of-the-fittest mentality. That's why you need to teach your toddler how to act appropriately and safely -- when you're around and when you're not. In a nutshell, your job is to implant a "good citizen" memory chip in her brain (Freud called this the superego) that will remind her how she's supposed to behave. It's a bit like breaking a wild horse, but you won't break your child's spirit if you do it

correctly. The seeds of discipline that you plant now will blossom later, and you'll be very thankful for the fruits of your labor. (Just don't expect a tree to grow overnight.) Here are the commandments you should commit to memory.

2. Expect rough spots. Certain situations and times of the day tend to trigger bad behavior. Prime suspect

number 1: transitions from one activity to the next (waking up, going to bed, stopping play to eat dinner). Give your child a heads-up so he's more prepared to switch gears ("After you build one more block tower, we will be having dinner").

2. Pick your battles. If you say no 20 times a day, it will lose its effectiveness. Prioritize behaviors into large, medium, and those too insignificant to bother with. In Starbucks terms, there are Venti, Grande, and Tall toddler screwups. If you ignore a minor infraction -- your toddler screams whenever you check your e-mail -- she'll eventually stop doing it because she'll see that it doesn't get a rise out of you.

3. Use a prevent defense. Sorry for the football cliche, but this one is easy. Make your house kid-friendly, and have reasonable expectations. If you clear your Swarovski crystal collection off the end table, your child

won't be tempted to fling it at the TV set. If you're taking your family out to dinner, go early so you won't have to wait for a table.

4. Make your statements short and sweet. Speak in brief sentences, such as "No hitting." This is much more effective than "Chaz, you know it's not nice to hit the dog." You'll lose Chaz right after "you know."

5. Distract and redirect. Obviously, you do this all day. But when you try to get your child interested in a different activity, she'll invariably go back to what she was doing -- just to see whether she can get away with it. Don't give up. Even if your child unrolls the entire toilet-paper roll for the 10th time today, calmly remove her from the bathroom and close the door.

6. Introduce consequences. Your child should learn the natural outcomes of his behavior -- otherwise known as cause and effect. For example, if he loudly insists on selecting his pajamas (which takes an eternity), then he's also choosing not to read books before bed. Cause: Prolonged picking = Effect: No time to read. Next time, he may choose his pj's more quickly or let you pick them out.

7. Don't back down to avoid conflict. We all hate to be the party pooper, but you shouldn't give in just to

escape a showdown at the grocery store. If you decide that your child can't have the cereal that she saw on TV, stick to your guns. Later, you'll be happy you did.

8. Anticipate bids for attention. Yes, your little angel will act up when your attention is diverted (making dinner, talking on the phone). That's why it's essential to provide some entertainment (a favorite toy, a quick snack). True story: My son once ate dog food while I was on the phone with a patient. Take-home lesson: If you don't provide something for your toddler to do when you're busy, she'll find something -- and the results may not be pretty.

9. Focus on the behavior, not the child. Always say that a particular behavior is bad. Never tell your child that he is bad. You want him to know that you love him, but you don't love the way he's acting right now.

10. Give your child choices. This will make her feel as if she's got a vote. Just make sure you don't offer too many options and that they're all things that

you want to accomplish, such as, "It's your choice: You can put your shoes on first, or your coat."

11. Don't yell. But change your voice. It's not the volume, but your tone that gets your point across. Remember The Godfather? Don Corleone never needed

to yell.

12. Catch your child being good. If you praise your child when he behaves well, he'll do it more often -- and he'll be less likely to behave badly just to get your attention. Positive reinforcement is fertilizer for that superego.

13. Act immediately. Don't wait to discipline your toddler. She won't remember why she's in trouble more than five minutes after she did the dirty deed.

14. Be a good role model. If you're calm under pressure, your child will take the cue. And if you have a temper tantrum when you're upset, expect that he'll do the same. He's watching you, always watching.

15. Don't treat your child as if she's an adult. She really doesn't want to hear a lecture from you and won't be able to understand it. The next time she throws her spaghetti, don't break into the "You Can't Throw Your Food" lecture. Calmly evict her from the kitchen for the night.

16. Use time-outs -- even at this age. Call it the naughty chair or whatever you like, but take your child away from playing and don't pay attention to him for one minute for each year of age. Depriving him of your attention is the most effective way to get your message across. Realistically, kids under 2 won't sit in a corner or

on a chair -- and it's fine for them to be on the floor kicking and screaming. (Just make sure the time-out location is a safe one.) Reserve time-outs for particularly inappropriate behaviors -- if your child bites his friend's arm, for example -- and use a time-out every time the offense occurs.

17. Don't negotiate with your child or make promises. This isn't Capitol Hill. Try to avoid saying anything like, "If you behave, I'll buy you that doll you want." Otherwise, you'll create a 3-year-old whose good behavior will always come with a price tag. (Think Veruca Salt from Charlie and the Chocolate Factory.)

18. Shift your strategies over time. What worked beautifully when your child was 15 months probably isn't going to work when he's 2. He'll have read your playbooks and watched the films.

19. Don't spank. Although you may be tempted at times, remember that you are the grown-up. Don't resort to acting like a child. There are many more effective ways of getting your message across. Spanking your child for hitting or kicking you, for example, just shows him that it's okay to use force. Finally, if your toddler is pushing your buttons for the umpteenth time and you think you're about to lose it, try to take a step back. You'll get a better idea of which manipulative behaviors your child is using and you'll get a fresh perspective on how to change your approach.

20. Remind your child that you love her. It's always good to end a discipline discussion with a positive comment. This shows your child that you're ready to move on and not dwell on the problem. It also reinforces the reason you're setting limits -- because you love her.

6.8 Disciplining Your Toddler to make the right choice

As a 2-year-old, Nathaniel Lampros of Sandy, Utah, was fascinated with toy swords and loved to duel with Kenayde, his 4-year-old sister. But inevitably, he'd whack her in the head, she'd dissolve in tears, and Angela, their mother, would come running to see what had happened. She'd ask Nathaniel to apologize, as well as give Kenayde a hug and make her laugh to pacify hurt feelings. If he resisted, Angela would put her son in time-out.

"I worried that Nathaniel would never outgrow his rough behavior, and there were days when I'd get so frustrated with him that I'd end up crying," recalls Lampros, now a mother of four. "But I really wanted Nathaniel to play

nicely, so I did my best to teach him how to do it." For many mothers, doling out effective discipline is one of the toughest and most frustrating tasks of parenting, a seemingly never-ending test of wills between you and your child. Because just when your 2-year-old "gets" that she can't thump her baby brother in the head with a doll, she'll latch on to another bothersome behavior — and the process starts anew.

How exactly does one "discipline" a toddler? Some people equate it with spanking and punishment, but that's not what we're talking about. As many parenting experts see it, discipline is about setting rules to stop your little one from engaging in behavior that's aggressive (hitting and biting), dangerous (running out in the street), and inappropriate (throwing food). It's also about following through with consequences when he breaks the rules — or what Linda Pearson, a Denver-based psychiatric nurse practitioner who specializes in family and parent counseling, calls "being a good boss." Here are seven strategies that can help you set limits and stop bad behavior.

1. Pick Your Battles

"If you're always saying, 'No, no, no,' your child will tune out the no and won't understand your priorities," says

Pearson, author of The Discipline Miracle. "Plus you can't possibly follow through on all of the nos.'" Define what's important to you, set limits accordingly, and follow through with appropriate consequences. Then ease up on little things that are annoying but otherwise fall into the "who cares?" category—the habits your child is likely to outgrow, such as insisting on wearing purple (and only purple).

"Keeping a good relationship with your child—who is of course in reality totally dependent upon you—is more important for her growth than trying to force her to respond in ways that she simply is not going to respond," says Elizabeth Berger, M.D., child psychiatrist and author of Raising Kids with Character. You may worry that "giving in" will create a spoiled monster, but Dr. Berger says this common anxiety isn't justified. For Anna Lucca of Washington, D.C., that means letting her 2-1/2-year-old daughter trash her bedroom before she dozes off for a nap. "I find books and clothes scattered all over the floor when Isabel wakes up, so she must get out of bed to play after I put her down," Lucca says. "I tell her not to make a mess, but she doesn't listen. Rather than try to catch her in the act and say,

'No, no, no,' I make her clean up right after her nap."

Lucca is also quick to praise Isabel for saying please and sharing toys with her 5-month-old sister. "Hopefully, the positive reinforcement will encourage Isabel to do more of the good behavior—and less of the bad," she says.

2. Know Your Child's Triggers Some misbehavior is preventable—as long as you can anticipate what will spark it and you create a game plan in advance, such as removing tangible temptations. This strategy worked for Jean Nelson of Pasadena, California, after her 2-year-old son took delight in dragging toilet paper down the hall, giggling as the roll unfurled behind

him. "The first two times Luke did it, I told him, 'No,' but when he did it a third time, I moved the toilet paper to a high shelf in the bathroom that he couldn't reach," Nelson says. "For a toddler, pulling toilet paper is irresistible fun. It was easier to take it out of his way than to fight about it."

If your 18-month-old is prone to grabbing cans off grocery store shelves, bring toys for him to play with in the cart while you're shopping. If your 2-year-old won't share her stuffed animals during playdates at home, remove them from the designated play area before her pal arrives. And if your 3-year-old likes to draw on the walls, stash the crayons in an out-of-reach drawer and don't let him color without supervision.

3. Practice Prevention

Some children act out when they're hungry, overtired, or frustrated from being cooped up inside, says Harvey Karp, M.D., creator of the DVD and book The Happiest Toddler on the Block. If your child tends to be happy and energetic in the morning but is tired and grumpy after lunch, schedule trips to the store and visits to the doctor for when she's at her best. Prepare her for any new experiences, and explain how you expect her to act. Also prepare her for shifting activities: "In a few minutes we'll need to pick up the toys and get ready to go home." The better prepared a child feels, the less likely she is to make a fuss.

4. Be Consistent

"Between the ages of 2 and 3, children are working hard to understand how their behavior impacts the people around them," says Claire Lerner, LCSW, director of parenting resources with Zero to Three, a nationwide nonprofit promoting the healthy development of babies and toddlers. "If your reaction to a situation keeps changing—one day you let your son throw a ball in the house and the next you don't—you'll confuse him with mixed signals." There's no timetable as to how many incidents and reprimands it will take before your child

stops a certain misbehavior. But if you always respond the same way, he'll probably learn his lesson after four or five times. Consistency was key for Orly Isaacson of Bethesda, Maryland, when her 18-month-old went through a biting phase. Each time Sasha chomped on Isaacson's finger, she used a louder-than-usual voice to correct her—"No, Sasha! Don't bite! That hurts Mommy!"—and then handed her a toy as a distraction. "I'm very low-key, so raising my voice startled Sasha and got the message across fast," she says. A caveat: by age 2, many kids learn how to make their parents lose resolve just by being cute. Don't let your child's tactics sway you—no matter how cute (or clever) they are.

5. Don't Get Emotional Sure, it's hard to stay calm when your 18-month-old yanks the dog's tail or your 3-year-old refuses to brush his teeth for the gazillionth night in a row. But if you scream in anger, the message you're trying to send will get lost and the situation will escalate, fast.

"When a child is flooded with a parent's negative mood, he'll see the emotion and won't hear what you're saying," advised the late William Coleman, M.D., professor of pediatrics at the University of North Carolina Medical School in Chapel Hill. Indeed, an angry reaction will only enhance the entertainment value for your child, so resist the urge to raise your voice. Take a deep breath, count to three, and get down to your child's eye level. Be fast and firm, serious and stern when you deliver the reprimand.

Trade in the goal of "controlling your child" for the goal of "controlling the situation," advises Dr. Berger. "This may mean re-adjusting your ideas of what is possible for a time until your daughter's self-discipline has a chance to grow a little more," she says. "You may need to lower your expectations of her patience and her self-control somewhat. If your goal is to keep the day going along smoothly, so that there are fewer opportunities for you both to feel frustrated, that would be a constructive direction."

6. Listen and Repeat

Kids feel better when they know they have been heard, so whenever possible, repeat your child's concerns. If she's whining in the grocery store because you won't let her open the cookies, say something like: "It sounds like you're mad at me because I won't let you open the cookies until we get home. I'm sorry you feel that way, but the store won't let us open things until they're paid

for. That's its policy." This won't satisfy her urge, but it will reduce her anger and defuse the conflict.

7. Keep It Short and Simple

If you're like most first-time parents, you tend to reason with your child when she breaks rules, offering detailed explanations about what she did wrong and issuing detailed threats about the privileges she'll lose if she doesn't stop misbehaving. But as a discipline strategy, overt-talking is as ineffective as becoming overly emotional, according to Dr. Coleman. While an 18-month-old lacks the cognitive ability to understand complex sentences, a 2- or 3-year-old with more developed language skills still lacks the attention span to absorb what you're saying.

Instead, speak in short phrases, repeating them a few times and incorporating vocal inflections and facial expressions. For example, if your 18-month-old swats your arm, say, "No, Jake! Don't hit Mommy! That hurts! No hitting." A 2-year-old can comprehend a bit more: "Evan, no jumping on the sofa! No jumping. Jumping is dangerous—you could fall. No jumping!" And a 3-year-old can process cause and effect, so state the consequences of the behavior: "Ashley, your teeth need to be brushed. You can brush them, or I can brush them

for you. You decide. The longer it takes, the less time we'll have to read Dr. Seuss."

8. Offer Choices

When a child refuses to do (or stop doing) something, the real issue is usually control: You've got it; she wants it. So, whenever possible, give your preschooler some control by offering a limited set of choices. Rather than commanding her to clean up her room, ask her, "Which would you like to pick up first, your books or your blocks?" Be sure the choices are limited, specific, and acceptable to you, however. "Where do you want to start?" may be overwhelming to your child, and a choice that's not acceptable to you will only amplify the conflict.

9. Watch Your Words

It helps to turn "you" statements into "I" messages. Instead of saying, "You're so selfish that you won't even share your toys with your best friend," try "I like it better when I see kids sharing their toys." Another good technique is to focus on do's rather than don'ts. If you tell a 3-year-old that he can't leave his trike in the hallway, he may want to argue. A better approach: "If you move your trike out to the porch, it won't get kicked and scratched so much." Make sure your tone and words do not imply that you no longer love your child. "I really

can't stand it when you act like that" sounds final; "I don't like it when you try to pull cans from the store shelves," however, shows your child that it's one specific behavior—not the whole person—that you dislike.

10. Teach Empathy

It's rarely obvious to a 3-year-old why he should stop doing something he finds fun, like biting, hitting, or grabbing toys from other children. Teach him empathy instead: "When you bite or hit people, it hurts them"; "When you grab toys away from other kids, they feel sad because they still want to play with those toys." This helps your child see that his behavior directly affects other people and trains him to think about consequences first.

11. Give a Time-Out

If repeated reprimands, redirection, and loss of privileges haven't cured your child of her offending behavior, consider putting her in time-out for a minute per year of age. "This is an excellent discipline tool for kids who are doing the big-time no-nos," Dr. Karp explains. Before imposing a time-out, put a serious look on your face and give a warning in a stern tone of voice ("I'm counting to three, and if you don't stop, you're going to time-out. One, two, THREE!"). If she doesn't

listen, take her to the quiet and safe spot you've designated for time-outs, and set a timer. When it goes off, ask her to apologize and give her a big hug to convey that you're not angry. "Nathaniel hated going to time-out for hitting his sister with the plastic sword, but I was clear about the consequences and stuck with it," says Angela Lampros. "After a few weeks, he learned his lesson." Indeed, toddlers don't like to be separated from their parents and toys, so eventually, the mere threat of a time-out should be enough to stop them in their tracks.

12. Talk Options

When you want your child to stop doing something, offer alternative ways for him to express his feelings: say, hitting a pillow or banging with a toy hammer. He needs to learn that while his emotions and impulses are acceptable, certain ways of expressing them are not. Also, encourage your child to think up his own options. Even 3-year-olds can learn to solve problems themselves. For instance, you could ask: "What do you think you could do to get Tiffany to share that toy with you?" The trick is to listen to their ideas with an open mind. Don't shoot down anything, but do talk about the consequences before a decision is made.

13. Reward Good Behavior

It's highly unlikely that your child will always do whatever you say. If that happened, you'd have to think about what might be wrong with her! Normal kids resist control, and they know when you're asking them to do something they don't want to do. They then feel justified in resisting you. In cases in which they do behave appropriately, a prize is like a spoonful of sugar: It helps the medicine go down. Judicious use of special treats and prizes is just one more way to show your child you're aware and respectful of his feelings. This, more than anything, gives credibility to your discipline demands.

14. Stay Positive

No matter how frustrated you feel about your child's misbehavior, don't vent about it in front of him. "If people heard their boss at work say, 'I don't know what to do with my employees. They run the company, and I feel powerless to do anything about it,' they'd lose respect for him and run the place even more," says Pearson. "It's the same thing when children hear their parents speak about them in a hopeless or negative way. They won't have a good image of you as their boss, and they'll end up repeating the behavior." Still, it's

perfectly normal to feel exasperated from time to time. If you reach that point, turn to your spouse, your pediatrician, or a trusted friend for support and advice. Ages & Stages Effective discipline starts with understanding where your child falls on the developmental spectrum. Our guide: At 18 months your child is curious, fearless, impulsive, mobile, and clueless about the consequences of her actions—a recipe for trouble. "My image of an 18-month-old is a child who's running down the hall away from his mother but looking over his shoulder to see if she's there and then running some more," said Dr. Coleman. "Though he's building a vocabulary and can follow simple instructions, he can't effectively communicate his needs or understand lengthy reprimands. He may bite or hit to register his displeasure or to get your attention. Consequences of misbehavior must be immediate. Indeed, if you wait even 10 minutes to react, he won't remember what he did wrong or tie his action to the consequence, says nurse practitioner Pearson.

At age 2 your child is using her developing motor skills to test limits, by running, jumping, throwing, and climbing. She's speaking a few words at a time, she becomes frustrated when she can't get her point across,

and she's prone to tantrums. She's also self-centered and doesn't like to share. Consequences should be swift, as a 2-year-old is unable to grasp time. But since she still lacks impulse control, give her another chance soon after the incident, says Lerner of Zero to Three.

At age 3 your child is now a chatterbox; he's using language to argue his point of view. Since he loves to be with other children and has boundless energy, he may have a tough time playing quietly at home. "Taking a 3-year-old to a gym or karate class will give him the social contact he craves and let him release energy," says Dr. Karp. "At this age, kids need that as much as they need affection and food." He also knows right from wrong, understands cause and effect, and retains information for several hours. Consequences can be delayed for maximum impact, and explanations can be more detailed. For example, if he hurls Cheerios at his sister, remind him about the no-food-throwing rule and explain that if he does it again, he won't get to watch Blues

Clues. If he continues to throw food, take it away from him. When he asks to watch TV, say, "Remember when

Mommy told you not to throw cereal and you did anyway? Well, the consequence is no Blues Clues today."

Chapter 7 Toddler timing and Developmental Milestones

Skills such as taking a first step, smiling for the first time, and waving "bye-bye" are called developmental milestones. Developmental milestones are things most children can do by a certain age. Children reach milestones in how they play, learn, speak, behave, and move (like crawling, walking, or jumping).

During the second year, toddlers are moving around more, and are aware of themselves and their surroundings. Their desire to explore new objects and people also is increasing. During this stage, toddlers will show greater independence; begin to show defiant behavior; recognize themselves in pictures or a mirror; and imitate the behavior of others, especially adults and older children. Toddlers also should be able to recognize the names of familiar people and objects, form simple phrases and sentences, and follow simple instructions and directions.

7.1 Positive Parenting Tips

Following are some of the things you, as a parent, can do to help your toddler during this time:Mother reading to toddler Read to your toddler daily. Ask her to find

objects for you or name body parts and objects. Play matching games with your toddler, like shape sorting and simple puzzles. Encourage him to explore and try new things. Help to develop your toddler's language by talking with her and adding to words she starts. For example, if your toddler says "baba", you can respond, "Yes, you are right—that is a bottle." Encourage your child's growing independence by letting him help with dressing himself and feeding himself. Respond to wanted behaviors more than you punish unwanted behaviors (use only very brief time outs). Always tell or show your child what she should do instead. Encourage your toddler's curiosity and ability to recognize common objects by taking field trips together to the park or going on a bus ride.

7.2 Child Safety First

Because your child is moving around more, he will come across more dangers as well. Dangerous situations can happen quickly, so keep a close eye on your child. Here are a few tips to help keep your growing toddler safe: Do NOT leave your toddler near or around water (for example, bathtubs, pools, ponds, lakes, whirlpools, or the ocean) without someone watching her. Fence off

backyard pools. Drowning is the leading cause of injury and death among this age group. Block off stairs with a small gate or fence. Lock doors to dangerous places such as the garage or basement. Ensure that your home is toddler proof by placing plug covers on all unused electrical outlets. Keep kitchen appliances, irons, and heaters out of reach of your toddler. Turn pot handles toward the back of the stove. Keep sharp objects such as scissors, knives, and pens in a safe place. Lock up medicines, household cleaners, and poisons. Do NOT leave your toddler alone in any vehicle (that means a car, truck, or van) even for a few moments. Store any guns in a safe place out of his reach. Keep your child's car seat rear-facing as long as possible. According to the National Highway Traffic Safety Administration, it's the best way to keep her safe. Your child should remain in a rear-facing car seat until she reaches the top height or weight limit allowed by the car seat's manufacturer. Once your child outgrows the rear-facing car seat, she is ready to travel in a forward-facing car seat with a harness.

7.3 The right Healthy Bodies for your Kids

Give your child water and plain milk instead of sugary

drinks. After the first year, when your nursing toddler is eating more and different solid foods, breast milk is still an ideal addition to his diet. Your toddler might become a very picky and erratic eater. Toddlers need less food because they don't grow as fast. It's best not to battle with him over this. Offer a selection of healthy foods and let him choose what she wants. Keep trying new foods; it might take time for him to learn to like them. Limit screen time and develop a media use plan for your family.external icon For children younger than 18 months of age, the AAP recommends that it's best if toddlers not use any screen media other than video chatting. Your toddler will seem to be moving continually—running, kicking, climbing, or jumping. Let him be active—he's developing his coordination and becoming strong. Make sure your child gets the recommended amount of sleep each night: For toddlers 1-2 years, 11–14 hours per 24 hours (including naps)

7.4 The proper height and Weight for your children

Baby growth charts for boys and girls are an important tool health providers use when it comes to comparing

your child's growth to other kids her age. But for the average parent, they can be a little confusing to decipher. To make it easier for you to get informed, we had experts breakdown the information you really want to know about your child's physical development. Here's a simple look at average height and weight growth at every age:

7.5 Baby Height and Weight Growth

Birth to 4 Days Old

The average newborn is 19.5 inches long and weighs 7.25 pounds. Boys have a head circumference of about 13.5 inches and girls measure in at 13.3 inches, according to the National Center for Health Statistics. A baby drops 5 to 10 percent of his total body weight in his first few days of life because of the fluid he loses through urine and stool, says Parents advisor Ari Brown, M.D., author of Baby 411.

5 Days to 3 Months

Babies gain about an ounce a day on average during this period, or half a pound per week, and they should be back to their birthweight by their second-week visit. Expect a growth surge around 3 weeks and then another one at 6 weeks.

3 Months to 6 Months

A baby should gain about half a pound every two weeks.

By 6 months, she should have doubled her birthweight.

7 Months to 12 Months

A child is still gaining about a pound a month. If you're nursing, your baby may not gain quite this much, or he may dip slightly from one percentile to another on the growth chart.

"At this point, babies may also burn more calories because they're starting to crawl or cruise," says Tanya Altmann, M.D., a Los Angeles pediatrician and author of Mommy Calls. Even so, by the time he reaches his first birthday, expect him to have grown 10 inches in length and tripled his birthweight and his head to have grown by about 4 inches.

Toddler Height and Weight Growth Age 1

Toddlers will grow at a slower pace this year but will gain about a half a pound a month and will grow a total of about 4 or 5 inches in height.

Age 2

A kid will sprout about 3 more inches by the end of her third year and will have quadrupled her birthweight by gaining about 4 more pounds. By now, your pediatrician

will be able to make a fairly accurate prediction about her adult height.

7.6 Preschooler Height and Weight Growth (Ages 3-4)

A preschooler will grow about 3 inches and gain 4 pounds each year. You may also find that your child starts to shed the baby fat from his face and looks lankier, since kids' limbs grow more by the time they are preschoolers, says Daniel Rauch, M.D., associate professor of pediatrics at Mount Sinai School of Medicine, in New York City.

7.7 Kids Height and Weight Growth (Ages 5+)

Starting at 5 years old, kids will begin to grow about 2 inches and gain 4 pounds each year until puberty (usually between 8 and 13 for girls and 10 and 14 for boys). Girls often reach their full height about two years after their first period. Boys usually hit their adult height around age 17.

7.8 How to keep your little toddler always happy and joyful

What Makes a Child Happy?

We all want the same things for our kids. We want them to grow up to love and be loved, to follow their dreams, to find success. Mostly, though, we want them to be happy. But just how much control do we have over our children's happiness?

Happy toddlers don't just happen...they're molded by parents who care! Bubbling giggles, chubby feet and colorful facial expressions all make-up a happy toddler!

It thrills my soul to see a content, obviously well-loved toddlers, explore their new world.

Their enthusiasm about daily life is contagious But some toddlers don't enjoy the blessings of a home that's filled with encouraging words, bundles of hugs and wheelbarrels full of kisses. Instead, they face daily criticism and harshness.

Have you ever heard a mother or father yell "Shut-up!" to their toddler? Unfortunately I have. I absolutely shutter and my teeth clench when I hear those anger-filled words. Instead of

tearing toddlers down, we should be encouraging them! Our focus should be creating happy toddlers — not creating sad, frustrated, misunderstood toddlers! I'll admit it. Sometimes it is crazy-easy to snap at toddler because you're trying to get other work done and they interrupt you once again. Be present in your toddler's life. Don't push your munchkin away when you are answering an email. Instead take a few moments and address her needs or wants. Take time to play with your toddler every day. Make tents together, color pictures, go on walks, bake together, try these simple toddler activities or whatever your child enjoys doing — do it! My youngest child enjoys swinging on our large patio swing. I try to make a "date" with him everyday for this special time. We are making memories! Set goals. Are you making dinner soon? Ask your toddler to help set the table. Do you clean your room in the morning? Ask your little one to help you make your bed. By giving toddlers responsibilities you are letting them know they have an important place in the family. When a child successfully completes a goal, like chores, he begins to develop security and an "I can do it!" attitude. It is my three-year-old son's task to open the door for visitors after they leave our home. He enjoys it so much! When he runs back to us, he always has an upbeat spirit and can't wait to help out in another area! Establish boundaries. Definite boundaries help a child understand what is acceptable in your home and what is not. If she does not know the rules, she can become paranoid and insecure of messing up. Make your rules reasonable and make sure you stick to them! If rules are not enforced, they are worthless.

Examples of acceptable rules for toddlers: λ No whining or screaming. λ Say "please" and "thank-you." λ Pick up your toys after you play.

λ Do not open the refrigerator. As your child obeys these rules, she will feel confident that she is able to obey "house ules." By establishing clear boundaries, you are promoting even more security for your toddler! Praise often. Criticism and negativity comes from everywhere in the outside world. Create a haven in your home by praising your toddler for jobs well-done, good attitudes or any positive characteristics you observe. Praising a child always adds extra dashes of happiness to the soul! Use eye contact. When praising or correcting, get down on your toddler's eye level and speak one-on-one together. You are letting him know she is the focus of your thoughts and energy. When he asks for a drink, squat down and ask him if he want juice or milk. Take these special short conversations to interact with your child in order to build his confidence in your unbiased love. Smile often. It's so easy to lose our smile when we're busy in daily tasks and life, isn't it? But a toddler finds much happiness in seeing a smile on mom's face. When a toddler sees that smile, the entire world seems like a peaceful, happy place...and the toddler knows that mom really does love and care for him! Our face speaks a thousand words! Listen. Nothing says, "You don't really matter," like someone not listening to what you are saying. When your toddler gets excited about something and wants to show and tell you about this new discovery, really listen and pay attention. Comment on their discovery. Don't just say, "Uh...yeah. That's neat. Now, go and play!" Your toddler knows when you're really listening and when you're just trying to shoo her away. Laugh!. Go ahead, let your hair down and be super silly with your toddler. Sing silly songs with them, talk in funny voices — anything to get a smile or laugh from your kiddos. Adding some silliness and fun to your toddler's day is the perfect way to build them up! Celebrate victories! Did your toddler finally get the potty-training deal?! :) Did your toddler learn to successfully and routinely nap?! Those are HUGE milestones and should be celebrated! Celebrate with just an ice cream cone, a trip to the park or some stickers! Keep it simple so it's always convenient to celebrate a new milestone in your munchkin's life. If your toddler is struggling with napping successfully, we have an awesome super-loaded course for that! Yay for a toddler naps ,right?!

Chapter 8 Montessori toddler discipline techniques

"The first idea that the child must acquire, in order to be actively disciplined, is that of the difference between good and evil; and the task of the educator lies in seeing that the child does not confound good with immobility, and evil with activity, as often happens in the case of the old-time discipline." Maria Montessori

A Montessori approach to discipline consists of a delicate balance between freedom and discipline. Like any part of Montessori education, it requires respect for the child.

I'd like to share some Montessori articles that give more insight into Montessori discipline, which by nature is a form of gentle/positive discipline. As a parent, your greatest ally is the child's own desire to grow, to learn, to master her own emotions, and to develop her own character. By keeping calm and respecting your child and her desires, you can help her on her own quest for inner discipline. By setting clear expectations and supporting your child's active thought and reflection, you can support the sense of personal autonomy she is naturally seeking as she follows her own unique path to physical, emotional, and intellectual independence.

8.1 Validate a child's emotions.

Of course, sometimes a child is going to want to take an action that is not permissible. A preschool-age child doesn't always understand why he is allowed to make some choices, but not others. Why can he choose what he has for dinner, but not when he has dinner? Why can he choose what to wear to school, but not whether he has to go to school in the first place? As an adult, you can help the child master himself in these frustrating moments by acknowledging his emotions. "You really wanted to wear your boots today! You are not in the mood for shoes! You're sad and mad about it." Be sure to allow your child time to experience the disappointment, and remember to save any reasoning or discussion until the initial emotion has run its course.

Montessori also encouraged teachers to talk with children about their behavior. To quote Dr. Montessori herself: .if he shows a tendency to misbehaves, she will check him with earnest words...

Many people misinterpret the Montessori method to be a permissive method that allows children unlimited freedom. In reality, the freedom is within limits that are carefully enforced through guidance by the teacher.

Common consequences in a Montessori classroom include:

λ Putting a material away that's not being used properly λ Cleaning up a mess or a spill

λ Staying close to the teacher

You can use these same consequences in your home. Natural Consequences

When it comes to discipline, parents often feel the need to impose consequences and punishments on the child, rather than letting things run their course. However, this teaches your child to fear getting caught by a parent, teacher or authority figure rather than learning the natural consequences of their actions.

But, what are natural consequences? In part, it's helping your child see what will happen as a result of their choices and actions, and letting it happen. Like what? For example, your child chooses to skip lunch. You allow them to skip lunch, but save their plate for later and when they ask for a snack, they can finish their lunch. Or your child leaves toys out and doesn't want to clean up. You can explain that leaving toys on the floor is dangerous for others because they might step on them and the family needs a clean place to live. Then, you can clean up the toys together, ensuring your

child helps. Rather than feeling threatened with punishment, your child learns to see how their actions affect themselves and others.

An easy way to implement this technique is by narrating what you see and helping your child predict the future. This also works well with aggressive behaviors like biting and hitting, and of course tantrums. You can say for example "I see you're angry. You want to hit me." However, in these cases, you may need to intervene to prevent children from getting hurt and say things like "I won't let you hurt your brother".

Montessori encouraged the use of control of error in materials and classroom activities. Natural consequences are the control of error of life. For example, Montessori encouraged the use of real glass dishes so that if children weren't careful or had an accident, the dishes would break. She believed this natural consequence was valuable for children to experience so that they could change their behavior in the future.

8.2 Best way to make your kids grow faster

Most parents would love for their children to be tall and strong, as it has been widely regarded as a sign of good health. Parents usually go to great lengths to ensure

that their children grow up healthily, and their height is treated as an indication of their overall health condition by most parts of the society.

Genes have the most say in determining the height of the child – however, it is not the only factor which influences it. Many external factors, like living conditions and a healthy diet, can influence the height of children quite a lot. Therefore, it is possible for parents to improve the chances of their children grow up to be tall and strong, through simple methods. Let us take a look at the top 10 ways to make your child grow taller.

8.3 How to Increase the Height of a Child

There are many ways a parent can influence the height of their child, and here's a list of the top ten ways.

1. A Balanced Diet

The most important aspect of how to increase your kid's height is to ensure that he gets proper nutrition. The food he consumes has to be healthy so that he grows up to be tall. A balanced diet has to include proteins, carbohydrates, fat and vitamins in the correct proportion – loading up on only one of these can have a detrimental effect. You must also ensure that the child keeps away from junk food most of the time – this includes food like

burgers, aerated sweetened drinks and fried items in general. Lean proteins have to be had aplenty, along with leafy vegetables and items rich in minerals like calcium and potassium. Simple carbs like pizza and cakes have to be avoided for the most part. Zinc has been found to have a huge effect on the growth of the child, so zinc-rich foods like squash seeds and peanuts must also be added to their diet. A balanced diet not only provides the right nutrients to increase your child's height but it will also make him stronger in every sense.

2. Stretching Exercises

Stretching exercises, even if they are simple ones, can have a huge impact on the height of your child. Introducing your child to stretching exercises from a

young age will facilitate the process of height growth. Stretching helps elongate the spine and also improves the posture of your child at all times. The exercises can be simple ones. Make him stand on his toes with his back against the wall and stretch the muscles in his leg while reaching up simultaneously. Another simple exercise for stretching involves the child sitting on the floor with his legs wide apart, and reaching to touch the toes of both legs with his arms. Stretching exercises to grow taller

3. Hanging

Hanging has been recommended for decades now, for parents who want their children to be taller. Hanging from bars also helps the spine elongate, which is an important part of becoming taller. Apart from regular hanging, you can also encourage your child to do pull-ups and chin-ups. Both make the muscles of the arm and the back stronger and are great exercises to help him keep fit.

4. Swimming

Swimming is another healthy habit, one which helps your child stay active and enjoy it, too. Swimming is a full-body exercise, meaning that it works all the muscles in the body to great effect. Swimming for a long time can help your child lose any extra fat present, making him healthier as a whole. The exercise involves a lot of stretching forward, which strengthens the spine and lays the groundwork for a tall, healthy body. Swimming is also a highly enjoyable activity- no child has ever said no to playing in the water!

5. Jogging

Jogging is an amazing exercise, not just for children- it has a range of benefits for grown-ups too. Jogging strengthens the bones in the leg and also increases the

quantity of HGH, the growth hormone, which is required for any growth in the body. To make it even more fun, you can maybe join in with your child and make jogging be an activity you do together!

6. Sleep

The importance of sleep can never be stressed upon enough, not just for children – for adults, too. Skipping sleep occasionally does not affect the growth of your child in the long term- however, you have to ensure that the child gets a good 8 hours of sleep on most nights, in order for him to be taller and stronger. This is because the growth hormone in children, HGH, is released only

when the child sleeps. This plays a direct role in making your child taller, so skipping sleep constantly is definitely a bad idea.

7. Posture

To increase your child's height, it is integral that he has a proper posture. Slumping or slouching can put unnecessary stress on the spine which can have many negative affects on the body. Additionally, poor posture can alter the shape of your child's spine which can compromise his growth. Make sure that your child practices good posture not only to increase his height but also to prevent any long term health issues. Remind

him to sit and stand up straight every time you see him slouching. There are many ways to make your child grow taller, but all of them work only when complemented by the other activities on the list. A good diet must be accompanied by regular exercise and sound sleep- else, you do not get what you want. Therefore, take care of your child the right way, and make him grow tall and strong.

8.4 How to keep your toddler busy and Happy at the same time

We all know that watching TV and playing video games isn't good for our kids. No parent is proud of how much time their kids spend in front of a screen but what are we supposed to do?

Sometimes, we just need to get things done. We need to clean the house or cook food or just take a few minutes for ourselves. It's hard to think of other things that could keep a kid distracted long enough to actually accomplish anything.

There are options, though. Sure, they take a bit more energy than just plopping a child in front of a screen, but encouraging your child to do something constructive just might be worth the extra effort.

We all know that watching TV and playing video games isn't good for our kids. No parent is proud of how much time their kids spend in front of a screen – but what are we supposed to do?

Sometimes, we just need to get things done. We need to clean the house or cook food or just take a few minutes for ourselves. It's hard to think of other things that could

keep a kid distracted long enough to actually accomplish anything. There are options, though. Sure, they take a bit more energy than just plopping a child in front of a screen, but encouraging your child to do something constructive just might be worth the extra effort.

Create a game box

Fill a box full of things your child can play with alone – things like coloring books, playing cards, or easy puzzles. When you need to keep your kids busy, give them the box. They might resist at first, but the more you do it, the more they'll accept "game box time" as part of their routine.

8.5 Have them make their own cartoon

Instead of watching cartoons, have your children make their own. Give them a piece of paper and some crayons, and ask them to draw you a hero and a bad

guy. When they're done, let them come back and tell you their hero's story.

8.6 Let them help you

If you're cooking or cleaning, let your kids help. Give them a job they can handle. For young kids, that might be stringing beans or setting the table. For older kids, that might be slicing vegetables, sweeping the house, or taking out the recycling.

8.7 Give them an important mission

Give your child a task, and make it a really big deal. Tell them they need to draw a picture for Dada, or that they need to make a block fort for Grandma. If they think it's an important job, they won't complain about working on it independently.

8.8 Generate an idea box

Brainstorm ideas with your children about what they can do to overcome boredom. Write down their suggestions, and put them in an empty box. Then, the next time they're bored, have them pick out one of their own suggestions. Given that it was their idea, they'll be more willing to actually do it.

8.9 Offer creative toys

Any toy that lets a child create is sure to keep them distracted for a long time. Invest in Legos, puzzles, and

Play-Dough. Not only will your child be able to play with them for hours, but they'll build up their spatial reasoning, too.

8.10 Design a treasure hunt

Hide something like a coin or a sticker somewhere in the house. Give your kids a clue, and let them run wild trying to find it. If you make it a bit tricky to find, you'll build up their resilience – and their ability to find things without begging for your help.

8.11 Let them play outside

Don't forget how your parents kept you busy. Just give your child a ball and a stick, and let them run wild. If you're worried about their safety, just keep them in sight of the window. They'll be fine.

8.12 Send them to a friend's house

Work out a deal with another parent on your street. When you need some time, send your kid over to play with their kid. To be fair, you'll have to let them send their kid over sometimes, too. When two kids play together, they keep themselves distracted.

8.13 Build a fort

Give your child a few pillows and a blanket, and challenge them to turn the couch into a fort. No child will turn down the chance to make a secret base – and they'll be much more likely to play independently once they're inside.

8.14 Make a sculpture

Give your child a few pipe cleaners and a piece of Styrofoam – or any other child-friendly items you might have on hand – and ask them to make a sculpture. Anything will do, but favorite heroes are a winning suggestion.

8.15 Listen to an audiobook

If your child's too young to read independently, pick up audio versions of their favorite books. Let them sit down and turn the pages while listening to a friendly voice read to them. Or, if you can't find a recording, use your phone to make one yourself. Play with locks and bolts Hand your child a lock and a key or a nut and bolt and let them play with it. Young kids, especially, will be mesmerized by the act of unlocking something – and they'll develop their motor skills while they're at it. Give them a mixed bag, and see if they can figure out which lock goes with which key.

Conclusion

Congratulations! You have made it to the end and I want to personally thank you for trusting us with this very important stage in your child's life. I want to wish you all the luck so that you are successful in potty training. You have taken the necessary steps that many have not. You have taken the steps to getting the information so that you know what you need to do to be successful.

Remember, you want to be consistent. Consistency is one of the most important things that you can do right now for your child to help them be successful in potty training. If there is anything that you learn from us today, please let that be that consistency is crucial. Secondly is the 'push.' Every time your child sits on that toilet, make sure they are pushing. Once they push they can get up even if they have not done anything on the toilet, as long as they have pushed it is okay for them to get up. Remember that you are in charge. You are the parent and you have to set the stage. You are pulling the strings, so remember that as your child is trying to push the boundaries you have set. As a parent and as a human this process maybe frustrating. This process maybe tough and we understand that, and so we're telling you to be parents and be human. You're

going to be frustrated, you're going to be mad, and you might even yell a couple times.

But don't let that keep you from saying to yourself, "I'm not a good parent." You are human, it's going to happen, so you have to be yourself and do how you normally do things and be yourself and be happy and true to yourself. Most importantly, as we said, get some rest because you don't want to be stressed during this process. You want to have as much energy as possible. That not only will increase the chances for your child success, but help you maintain your sanity and increase your own success as well. We wish you good luck and lots of fun. Be strong!

CPSIA information can be obtained
at www.ICGtesting.com
Printed in the USA
BVHW011443080421
604344BV00006BA/256